Memory Boosting Activities for Seniors

Enhance Mental Agility and Quality of Life with Engaging Puzzles, Cognitive Games, and Strategies for Improved Daily Functioning

H. J. Marks

Disclaimer

Dear Reader,

I am excited to start this cognitive journey with you. But before we begin, it is important to note that this book primarily serves as a guide and informational resource, providing insights into the world of memory games and their benefits for seniors.

However, I want to be transparent about the nature of the content within these pages. This book does not include specific exercises or techniques for memory improvement. Instead, we have curated a rich collection of memory-enhancing exercises and techniques accessible through URLs provided within the text.

To fully experience the array of memory games and exercises at your disposal, we encourage you to visit the provided URLs. There, you will find a wealth of resources and activities designed to stimulate and challenge your cognitive abilities. Feel free to explore and engage with as many exercises as you wish to create a personalized and enjoyable memory-enhancement experience.

Please be advised that individual results may vary, and it is always recommended to consult with a healthcare professional before starting any new cognitive activities, especially for individuals with pre-existing medical conditions.

Wishing you a fulfilling and mentally engaging journey toward improved memory and cognitive well-being.

Table of Contents

Introduction

In life, memories are the threads that weave our experiences into a rich and meaningful narrative. As we embark on the golden journey of our senior years, preserving and enhancing our cognitive abilities becomes an essential pursuit. The concern about memory loss is a sentiment shared by many seniors, but fear not, for within these pages, a delightful exploration of memory games awaits you.

This book is not just a manual; it is a companion for those who wish to engage in activities that not only safeguard their memories but also infuse joy into their daily lives. Whether you find yourself concerned about memory loss or simply yearning to sharpen your cognitive prowess, you have embarked on a journey that promises to be both enlightening and entertaining.

In the later years of life, there is a profound desire to savor the moments and experiences that have shaped our existence. Memories, like precious treasures, provide a glimpse into the tapestry of our lives. However, the fear of memory loss can cast a shadow over these golden years. It is this concern, coupled with the innate human desire for continuous growth and learning, that has inspired the creation of this book.

Memories are the soul's imprints—the stories that define who we are. As seniors, we stand at the intersection of a lifetime of experiences, and the preservation of these memories becomes a celebration of our unique journey.

Memory, much like a garden, requires care and attention. Just as a gardener tends to the soil, cultivating an environment for vibrant growth, we too can nurture our memories. This book becomes a toolkit for cultivating the garden of your mind, allowing the blossoms of recollection to flourish.

As we navigate the complexities of aging, it is crucial to approach the preservation and enhancement of our cognitive abilities with a sense of curiosity and optimism. The pages that follow are not a prescription for staving off the inevitable passage of time but rather an invitation to embrace the present moment and the incredible potential that resides within our minds.

For those who may harbor concerns about memory loss, rest assured that this book is not intended to be a clinical dissertation on the complexities of neurobiology. Instead, it is a friendly conversation about the power of play, the joy of learning, and the benefits of engaging in activities designed to stimulate the mind.

Within these pages, you will discover a world where memory becomes an ally, not an adversary. Memory games, far from being just exercises, are portrayed as the tools of a grand adventure—a journey into the realms of cognition where fun and mental fitness coexist harmoniously.

In the pursuit of memory enhancement, the marriage of fun and learning becomes the cornerstone. Each game is a note, contributing to the harmonious melody of mental stimulation. From word associations that tickle your linguistic prowess to spatial puzzles that dance with your visual memory, every game is designed to make the learning process an exhilarating experience.

The essence of this book is to infuse joy into the act of preserving and sharpening your cognitive abilities. It is not about grueling tasks or tedious drills; it is about creating an atmosphere where laughter and learning intertwine, fostering an environment that is conducive to mental flourishing.

As we engage in memory games, it is worth taking a moment to appreciate the science behind the play. The brain, a marvel of nature, thrives on novelty and challenge. These games act as sparks, igniting neural pathways and promoting neuroplasticity—the brain's remarkable ability to adapt and reorganize itself. Through play, we tap into the brain's inherent plasticity, sculpting it into a resilient and agile masterpiece.

The science is not a dry set of principles; rather, it is the magical wand that turns each game into a transformative experience. It is the reason why a simple card-matching activity can become a gateway to heightened memory recall, and a crossword puzzle can serve as a secret passage to linguistic enrichment.

One of the great misconceptions about aging is the notion that mental decline is inevitable. This book aims to shatter that stereotype. Seniors are not passive observers of their cognitive destiny; they are active participants in shaping the trajectory of their mental well-being.

Games for seniors are not a concession to aging; they are a rebellion against stagnation. They embody the spirit of continuous growth and the belief that the mind, like fine wine, can improve with time. By breaking free from stereotypes, we embrace a mindset that fosters resilience and cultivates a positive approach to aging.

Before delving into the myriad of games awaiting you, understanding the foundational strategies is essential. These strategies serve as the warp and weft of the cognitive tapestry you are about to weave.

Visualization, the art of creating vivid mental images, becomes a painter's brush on the canvas of memory. Association, the linking of ideas and concepts, forms the connective tissue that strengthens neural connections. These are not abstract concepts; they are tools you wield in the journey toward enhanced memory.

With the foundation set and the strategies in hand, it is time to embark on this odyssey. Each game is an island, waiting to be explored, with challenges and treasures unique to its landscape.

From the simplicity of matching games that exercise your recall to the complexity of strategic games that test your problem-solving abilities, the voyage promises a diverse and enriching experience. It is not about the destination; it is about the journey and the discoveries made along the way.

As you turn the pages of this book and immerse yourself in the world of memory games, remember that this journey is a rediscovery—a rediscovery of the joy inherent in learning, the resilience of the mind, and the limitless potential residing within you.

So, dear reader, let the games begin. May each game be a stepping stone in your quest for mental vitality, and may the laughter that accompanies the challenges be the soundtrack to your memory's triumphs. Embrace the adventure, revel in the play, and may the chapters of your senior years be written with the ink of newfound memories and unwavering cognitive strength.

Whether you are here with a genuine concern about memory loss or simply seeking to add a dash of excitement to your daily routine, welcome. Welcome to a space where age is but a number, and the mind is an ever-evolving landscape ready to be explored. The journey ahead promises laughter, challenges, and, above all, the sheer delight of discovering the untapped potential within the recesses of your memory.

Chapter 1:

Understanding Memory Loss

Memories are not fixed or frozen but are transformed, disassembled, reassembled, and recategorized with every act of recollection. –Oliver Sacks

Before we delve into the realms of memory enhancement and cognitive well-being, it is crucial to unravel the complexities of memory loss. Only by comprehending what memory loss is (and what it is not), identifying its origins, and recognizing its potential impact, can we begin to navigate the path toward cognitive resilience.

Memory loss is a topic that often sparks worry and curiosity in equal measure. As we age, questions about forgetfulness, lapses in recall, and the overall health of our cognitive faculties become more prevalent. It is essential to approach this subject with both an inquisitive mind and a proactive spirit. In this chapter, we will embark on a journey together to demystify memory loss, shedding light on its various facets and providing you with the tools to take the first steps toward managing it effectively.

We will explore memory, understanding its nuances, and differentiating normal age-related forgetfulness from more serious cognitive concerns. By grasping the roots of memory loss, we empower ourselves to make informed decisions about our cognitive health. It is not about dwelling on what might be slipping away but rather about embracing the knowledge that will enable us to maintain and enhance our cognitive capacities.

Here, you will discover the science behind memory, its workings, and the factors that contribute to its ebb and flow. Together, we will explore how memory loss can manifest and the various ways it can impact our daily lives. Armed with this knowledge, you will be better equipped to embark on the journey of memory enhancement and cognitive well-being with confidence and enthusiasm.

Unveiling the Origins of Memory Loss

Memory loss, especially in the senior years, can stem from various sources, ranging from natural aging processes to more complex medical conditions. That is why we will delve into why memory loss occurs, exploring both disease-related and non-disease-related causes that are pertinent to seniors.

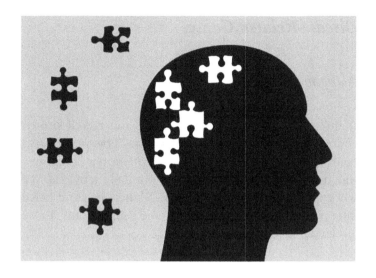

Natural Aging Processes

The passage of time inevitably brings changes to our bodies, and our brains are no exception. As we age, there is a natural decline in certain cognitive functions, including memory. The brain undergoes subtle structural alterations, such as reduced blood flow and changes in the communication between neurons.

These age-related changes can affect memory retrieval and processing speed. Understanding these normal age-related shifts is crucial for distinguishing them from more concerning forms of memory loss.

Disease-Related Causes

Alzheimer's Disease

Alzheimer's disease is perhaps the most well-known contributor to memory loss in seniors. This progressive neurological disorder affects memory, cognitive functions, and the ability to carry out daily activities. We will explore the characteristics of Alzheimer's and delve into strategies for managing and supporting those affected.

Vascular Dementia

Vascular dementia results from impaired blood flow to the brain, often due to strokes or other vascular conditions. It can lead to memory loss and cognitive decline, and we will discuss preventive measures and lifestyle choices that can mitigate its impact.

Mild Cognitive Impairment (MCI)

MCI is an intermediate stage between normal age-related cognitive decline and more severe conditions like Alzheimer's disease. Understanding MCI is crucial as it can provide an opportunity for early intervention and lifestyle adjustments.

Non-Disease-Related Causes

Medication Side Effects

Some medications commonly prescribed to seniors may have side effects that impact memory. We will explore how to navigate the balance between medication management and cognitive well-being.

Stress and Depression

Emotional well-being plays a significant role in cognitive health. Chronic stress and depression can contribute to memory issues, and we will discuss strategies for maintaining mental and emotional balance.

Nutritional Deficiencies

Proper nutrition is vital for brain health. We will examine how deficiencies in essential nutrients like vitamin B12 and omega-3 fatty acids can affect memory and cognition.

By unraveling the various causes of memory loss, we empower ourselves to take proactive steps in managing and enhancing our cognitive abilities.

Decoding the Neuroscience of Memory Loss

Understanding the science behind memory loss involves unraveling the fascinating processes that occur within our cranial command center.

Neurons and Synapses

At the heart of memory is the dance of neurons and synapses. Neurons are the brain's messengers, communicating through tiny gaps called synapses. When we learn something new or experience an event, neurons fire, creating connections in the form of synapses. These connections encode information, creating the foundation for memories.

Hippocampus

Think of the hippocampus as your brain's librarian. Nestled deep within, this seahorse-shaped structure plays a pivotal role in forming and retrieving memories. It acts as a sorting center, helping organize information into short-term and long-term storage.

Formation of Memories

Memories are not static; they undergo a complex process of encoding, consolidation, and retrieval. When we learn something, neural circuits are activated, and the information is temporarily stored in the hippocampus. With repetition and relevance, these memories move to long-term storage in various regions of the brain.

The Role of Neurotransmitters

Neurotransmitters, the brain's chemical messengers, play a crucial role in memory function. Acetylcholine, for instance, enhances attention and learning. Imbalances in neurotransmitters can disrupt these processes, contributing to memory issues.

Amygdala and Emotion

The amygdala, an almond-shaped structure, adds an emotional flavor to memories. Events tied to strong emotions are often better remembered. Understanding the interplay between emotion and memory sheds light on why certain memories stand out more vividly.

The Impact of Aging

As we age, the brain changes. The prefrontal cortex, responsible for decision-making and multitasking, may experience a decline. Blood flow and neurotransmitter levels may fluctuate. The hippocampus may show signs of wear and tear. These natural aging processes contribute to the nuances of age-related memory changes.

Neuroplasticity

The brain's remarkable ability to adapt and reorganize itself is known as neuroplasticity. Despite challenges, the brain can form new connections, compensating for age-related changes. Engaging in activities that stimulate neuroplasticity becomes a key strategy in supporting cognitive health.

The Impact of Memory Loss

Memory loss can manifest in subtle ways, and understanding these signs is a crucial step in proactive cognitive care. Let us take a look at various indicators, shedding light on the nuances that distinguish ordinary forgetfulness from more significant memory concerns.

Common Signs of Memory Loss

- **Forgetfulness in Routine Tasks:** Everyday activities, such as forgetting to turn off the stove, misplacing keys, or missing appointments, may signal memory lapses. If these instances become frequent and disrupt daily life, they warrant attention.

- **Repetitive Questions or Statements:** Individuals experiencing memory loss may ask the same questions repeatedly or make the same statements, unaware of having done so. This repetition can be a red flag for memory-related challenges.

- **Difficulty in Recalling Names and Faces:** Struggling to remember names, especially of people one has known for a while, can be a sign of memory issues. This extends to difficulty recognizing familiar faces or places.

- **Misplacing Items in Unusual Locations:** Putting items in unusual places and then having difficulty locating them is a classic sign of memory lapses. For example, finding keys in the refrigerator or a wallet in the bathroom.

- **Confusion in Time and Place:** Memory loss can lead to confusion about the current date, day of the week, or even the year. Misunderstanding or forgetting appointments and events becomes more noticeable.

- **Decreased Ability to Learn New Information:** Difficulty grasping and retaining new information, whether it is a simple conversation or a new skill, may indicate memory challenges.

- **Struggling With Familiar Tasks:** Memory loss can impact one's ability to perform routine tasks, such as following a recipe, operating household appliances, or managing finances.

It is crucial to note that occasional forgetfulness is a natural part of aging, and not every instance should raise an alarm. However, when these signs become consistent, affect daily life, and cause distress, seeking professional guidance is advisable. Memory loss can stem from various factors, including medical conditions, stress, or lifestyle choices.

By understanding the impact of memory loss and recognizing its signs, we empower ourselves to take proactive steps toward a vibrant and resilient cognitive future.

The Daily Influence of Memory Loss

In the realm of memory loss, it is crucial to comprehend its daily impacts, especially in the realms of emotions, relationships, work, and personal hygiene.

Memory loss extends beyond forgetfulness; it shapes our daily experiences and interactions.

Emotional Impact

Memory loss can evoke a range of emotions, both for the individuals experiencing it and their loved ones. Frustration, anxiety, and a sense of loss may surface as daily tasks become more challenging. Understanding and acknowledging these emotions is a vital step in coping with the emotional impact of memory loss.

Relationship Dynamics

The world of our relationships is intricately created with shared memories and experiences. Memory loss can strain these connections as familiar stories become forgotten, and shared histories may need to be revisited. Communication may require adjustments, and patience becomes a precious commodity. However, fostering understanding and finding joy in the present moment can help navigate these changes, strengthening the bonds with those we hold dear.

Work Challenges

For individuals still engaged in work or professional pursuits, memory loss can present unique challenges. Forgetfulness during meetings, difficulty in recalling important details, or struggling with tasks that once seemed routine can impact one's professional confidence. Strategies to manage these challenges, such as effective note-taking and organization, become essential for maintaining productivity and workplace harmony.

Personal Hygiene and Self-Care

Memory loss can influence personal hygiene and self-care routines. Forgetting whether one has taken medication, neglecting dental care, or facing challenges in maintaining personal grooming habits are common concerns. Establishing daily routines, utilizing reminders, and enlisting the support of caregivers or loved ones can contribute to maintaining a sense of personal well-being.

Dispelling Misconceptions About Memory Loss

Misunderstandings can lead to unnecessary worry and hinder proactive steps toward cognitive well-being. Let us unravel 10 common misconceptions, providing a more realistic view of memory loss for a clearer understanding.

1. **Forgetfulness Equals Alzheimer's:** Contrary to popular belief, occasional forgetfulness does not automatically indicate Alzheimer's disease.

Normal age-related forgetfulness is common and distinct from more serious cognitive conditions.

2. **Memory Loss Is Inevitable With Aging:** While some cognitive decline may occur with age, severe memory loss is not an inevitable consequence of getting older. Many seniors maintain sharp cognitive abilities well into their later years.

3. **Memory Loss Is Always Permanent:** Memory loss is not always permanent. In some cases, memory issues can be reversible, especially when related to medication side effects, stress, or nutritional deficiencies.

4. **Only Older Adults Experience Memory Loss:** Memory loss is not exclusive to seniors. Younger individuals can also experience memory challenges due to stress, lifestyle factors, or medical conditions.

5. **There Is Nothing You Can Do to Prevent Memory Loss:** On the contrary, adopting a healthy lifestyle, engaging in cognitive activities, and managing stress can contribute significantly to cognitive health. Proactive measures can make a difference.

6. **Memory Loss Means Total Memory Failure:** Memory loss often manifests as forgetfulness in specific areas rather than a complete memory wipe. Individuals may have difficulty recalling

names, but other aspects of memory remain intact.

7. **Memory Loss Only Affects Cognitive Abilities:** The impact of memory loss extends beyond cognitive functions. It can influence emotional well-being, relationships, and daily activities, highlighting the holistic nature of cognitive health.

8. **Memory Loss Is Always a Sign of Serious Illness:** While memory loss can be associated with serious conditions like Alzheimer's, it can also result from stress, anxiety, or depression. Not every instance of forgetfulness is a cause for alarm.

9. **Memory Exercises Guarantee Immunity:** Engaging in memory exercises is beneficial, but they do not guarantee immunity against memory loss. A holistic approach, including a healthy lifestyle and social engagement, is essential.

10. **Ignoring Memory Issues Makes Them Go Away:** Ignoring memory issues does not make them disappear. Early acknowledgment, seeking professional advice, and adopting proactive strategies are key to managing and improving cognitive health.

Understanding Learning Styles and Memory

Each of us has a unique approach to acquiring and retaining information, and understanding our learning style can significantly impact our ability to enhance cognitive function.

Learning styles refer to the preferred ways individuals absorb, process, and retain information. These preferences can influence how we engage with new concepts, skills, and experiences. Recognizing and embracing our learning style can be a powerful tool in optimizing memory and cognitive function.

Identifying your learning style is a self-reflective process. Consider past learning experiences where you felt exceptionally engaged and retained information well. Was it through visual aids, verbal explanations, hands-on activities, or reading and writing? Pay attention to your study habits, observing if you naturally gravitate toward reading, listening, interacting with material, or a combination of these. Reflect on your hobbies and how you naturally approach and learn within those activities.

Visual learners grasp information best through visual aids such as diagrams, charts, and images. Auditory learners thrive on verbal communication and benefit from listening to information. Kinesthetic learners learn best through hands-on experiences and physical activities. Reading/Writing learners absorb information most effectively through reading and writing.

Experiment with different methods to identify your learning style. Try incorporating various approaches into your routine and observe which methods feel most effective. By understanding your learning style, you can tailor your learning experience to optimize memory retention and cognitive engagement.

The Influence of Learning Styles on Memory

Our unique ways of absorbing and processing information play an important role in how effectively we remember and retain new knowledge. Let us unravel the direct influence of learning styles on memory and how understanding this connection can pave the way for a more personalized and effective cognitive journey.

- **Visual Learners:** For visual learners, the use of charts, diagrams, and visual aids can significantly enhance memory. Associating information with images and spatial arrangements creates a robust memory imprint.

- **Auditory Learners:** Auditory learners benefit from verbal explanations, discussions, and listening to information. Utilizing podcasts and lectures, and engaging in conversations can enhance memory recall for individuals with this learning style.

- **Kinesthetic Learners:** Kinesthetic learners, who thrive on hands-on experiences, may find that physically engaging with information through activities, experiments, or interactive exercises fosters better memory retention.

- **Reading/Writing Learners:** Individuals with a reading/writing learning style often excel in memory when they read and take notes. Translating information into written form and revisiting written notes can reinforce memory for this group.

Understanding your learning style allows you to tailor memory enhancement strategies to your individual preferences. By aligning memory activities with your preferred way of learning, you can create a more effective and enjoyable approach to cognitive well-being.

In the chapters that follow, I will provide a diverse array of memory enhancement activities and strategies meticulously designed to cater to all learning styles. Whether you identify as a visual, auditory, kinesthetic, or reading/writing learner, this book is your guide to a vibrant cognitive future.

I aim to offer you a personalized and enjoyable journey toward memory enhancement. By embracing activities aligned with your unique learning style, you will not only boost your memory but also foster a deeper connection with the joy of learning.

In summary, this chapter has shed light on the diverse causes and impacts of memory loss, debunked common misconceptions, and explored the profound influence of learning styles on memory enhancement. Understanding these facets is essential within our broader framework of cognitive empowerment, as I strive to provide seniors with a comprehensive toolkit for memory improvement. As we pivot toward the next chapter, we will delve into the prevalence of memory loss, offering insights that lay the foundation for the subsequent exploration of proven strategies and engaging activities designed to enhance cognitive resilience. Join me on this journey as we unravel the prevalence of memory loss and chart a course toward a more vibrant and enriched cognitive future.

Chapter 2:

Memory Loss Prevalence

We didn't realize we were making memories, we just knew we were having fun. –Winnie the Pooh

In the landscape of concerns that accompany aging, the worry of memory loss stands out as a common and formidable challenge for many seniors. It is a subject that often carries with it a cloud of misconceptions and fears, leaving people uncertain about the prevalence of memory-related issues and the effectiveness of preventative measures. In this chapter, we embark on a journey to dispel those misconceptions, providing you with a clear understanding of just how prevalent memory loss is among seniors. More importantly, we will explore proven and enjoyable methods to enhance cognitive function, ensuring that whether you are already experiencing memory challenges or simply seeking to be proactive, the strategies outlined here will work for you. So, let us delve into the facts, erase any lingering doubts, and empower you to embrace a future where a sharp and vibrant memory is not only possible but within your reach.

Does Everyone Experience Memory Loss?

No, they do not.

Contrary to popular belief, memory decline is not an inevitable part of the aging process. Many seniors maintain sharp and vibrant memories well into their golden years, and this chapter is dedicated to ensuring that you are one of them.

The prevalence of memory loss among seniors varies, and it is essential to understand that not everyone encounters significant memory challenges. In fact, research made by Hwang, Park & Kim (2018) suggests that individuals who actively engage in activities to protect their memory are more likely to maintain cognitive vitality.

It is important to distinguish between normal memory problems and those that may be cause for concern. Normal memory lapses, such as momentarily forgetting a name or misplacing keys, are common occurrences that happen to people of all ages. These minor forgetfulness instances are often related to stress, fatigue, or distractions, and they do not necessarily indicate a decline in cognitive function.

On the other hand, age-related memory concerns involve more persistent and noticeable issues. For instance, consistently forgetting important appointments, struggling to recall familiar faces or places, or experiencing challenges in performing routine tasks may be indicators of more significant cognitive changes. Recognizing these distinctions is vital in gauging whether your memory experiences fall within the normal spectrum or if they require closer attention.

Signs You Might Experience Memory Loss

While these indicators do not guarantee memory decline, they serve as noteworthy signals that warrant attention and proactive measures. Here are some signs to consider:

- **Forgetfulness Impacting Daily Life:** If you find that forgetfulness is increasingly affecting your daily activities, such as forgetting to turn off appliances, missing appointments, or frequently misplacing essential items, it may be a signal to pay closer attention to your cognitive health.

- **Difficulty in Learning and Retaining New Information:** Struggling to grasp and remember new information could be an early sign of memory challenges. If you notice a decline in your ability to absorb and retain fresh knowledge, it is essential to explore strategies to enhance your memory.

- **Repetitive Questions or Statements:** If you find yourself asking the same questions or making the same statements repeatedly, it might be an indicator of memory lapses. Pay attention to patterns of repetition, as they can highlight areas for improvement in memory function.

- **Confusion With Time or Place:** Losing track of time or becoming disoriented about your location can be concerning signs. If you frequently forget appointments or struggle to recall where you are, it is crucial to investigate the root causes and address them proactively.

- **Difficulty in Problem-Solving:** Memory loss can also impact your ability to solve problems or make decisions. If you notice challenges in reasoning or finding solutions to everyday issues, it is worth exploring ways to sharpen your cognitive skills.

- **Social Withdrawal or Changes in Personality:** Memory decline can sometimes manifest in changes in social behavior or personality. If you or your loved ones observe shifts in your social interactions, mood, or personality, it is essential to consider potential cognitive implications.

It is crucial to note that experiencing one or more of these signs does not automatically mean you will lose your memory in the future. Many factors contribute to cognitive health, and these signs are simply indicators that merit attention and proactive measures. Remember, being aware of these signs is the first step toward taking charge of your cognitive health and enjoying a vibrant, sharp memory in the years to come.

Stages of Memory Loss

Memory loss, like many age-related conditions, often progresses through distinct stages, each marked by varying levels of severity and impact on daily life. Understanding these stages is crucial for seniors who are concerned about their cognitive well-being or those looking to enhance their memory capacity. Let us delve into the common stages of memory loss:

- **Normal Age-Related Forgetfulness:** The earliest stage is characterized by what is considered normal, age-related forgetfulness. This includes occasional lapses in memory, such as forgetting names, misplacing keys, or blanking on minor details. These forgetful moments are generally sporadic, do not significantly interfere with daily life, and are often dismissed as part of the natural aging process.

- **Mild Cognitive Impairment (MCI):** As mentioned in the previous chapter, MCI represents a noticeable increase in forgetfulness beyond typical age-related occurrences. Individuals with MCI may experience challenges in remembering recent events, names, or important details. While these difficulties may not yet significantly impact daily functioning, they are more pronounced than what is considered typical for one's age.

- **Early Stage Memory Loss:** The early stages of memory loss, often associated with conditions like Alzheimer's disease, involve more pronounced cognitive challenges. Memory loss extends beyond occasional forgetfulness, affecting the ability to recall recent conversations, remember appointments, or maintain organization. At this stage, individuals may also struggle with problem-solving and exhibit changes in mood or personality.

- **Moderate Memory Loss:** As memory loss progresses, the moderate stage involves a substantial decline in cognitive function. People may have difficulty recognizing familiar faces, forget significant details about their personal history, and experience challenges with daily tasks such as dressing or cooking. Communication skills may also be affected, and supervision and assistance may become necessary.

- **Severe Memory Loss (Advanced Dementia):** In the advanced stages of memory loss, people may lose the ability to communicate coherently, recognize loved ones, or perform basic self-care tasks. The impact on daily life becomes profound, requiring constant support and care. Advanced dementia is often associated with significant changes in brain structure and function.

It is important to note that these stages are generalizations, and the progression of memory loss can vary widely among individuals. Some may remain in the mild cognitive impairment stage for an extended period, while others may experience a more rapid decline. Additionally, the causes of memory loss can differ, ranging from Alzheimer's disease to vascular dementia or other underlying health conditions. Remember, knowledge is a powerful tool in navigating the complexities of memory loss, and with the right approach, one can maintain cognitive vitality and enjoy a fulfilling and active lifestyle.

Preventative Success: Empowering Your Memory Journey

In the realm of cognitive health, the question often arises: Can memory loss truly be prevented, or are we destined to succumb to the inevitable decline that comes with aging? The good news is that the narrative is far from predetermined. Research and real-life success stories underscore the notion that with the right strategies, commitment, and a dash of enthusiasm, you can actively work to prevent memory loss or, at the very least, significantly reduce your risk (LaMotte, 2023).

The Power of Lifestyle Choices

The first cornerstone of preventative success lies in the realm of lifestyle choices. Our daily habits and routines exert a profound influence on the health of our brain and, consequently, our memory. Consider the following lifestyle factors that have been linked to cognitive health:

- **Regular Physical Exercise:** Engaging in regular physical activity has been consistently associated with a reduced risk of cognitive decline. Exercise not only improves blood flow to the brain but also stimulates the growth of new neurons, enhancing cognitive function. Activities such as brisk walking, swimming, or even gardening can contribute significantly to maintaining a healthy brain.

- **Nutrient-Rich Diet:** The adage "You are what you eat" holds particular relevance when it comes to cognitive health. A diet rich in antioxidants, omega-3 fatty acids, and other essential nutrients provides the building blocks for a resilient brain. Incorporate colorful fruits, vegetables, whole grains, and fatty fish into your meals to nourish your brain and support cognitive function.

- **Mental Stimulation:** Keeping your brain active and engaged is a powerful tool in preventing memory loss. Activities that challenge your cognitive abilities, such as puzzles, games, reading, or learning a new skill, promote the formation of new neural connections. Think of your brain as a muscle—the more you use it, the stronger and more resilient it becomes.

- **Quality Sleep:** Adequate and restful sleep is a critical component of cognitive health. During sleep, the brain consolidates memories and clears out toxins that accumulate during waking hours. Establishing a consistent sleep routine and creating a comfortable sleep environment are essential for supporting memory and overall brain function.

- **Stress Management:** Chronic stress has been linked to cognitive decline, making stress management a crucial aspect of preventative strategies. Practices such as meditation, deep breathing exercises, and hobbies that bring joy and relaxation can help mitigate the impact of stress on your brain.

The Role of Social Connection

Human beings are inherently social creatures, and the power of social connections should not be underestimated in the quest for memory preservation. Research made by Umberson & Montez (2010) consistently shows that maintaining strong social ties can have a protective effect on cognitive health.

- **Meaningful Relationships:** Cultivating and sustaining meaningful relationships with family, friends, and community members contributes to emotional well-being and cognitive resilience. Engage in social activities, join clubs, or volunteer to foster a sense of connection and purpose.

- **Intellectual Stimulation Through Social Interaction:** Social interactions provide an intellectually stimulating environment, challenging your brain in unique ways. Engage in conversations, participate in group activities, and share experiences to keep your mind active and agile.

The Mind-Body Connection

The mind and body are intricately connected, and a holistic approach to preventative measures takes into account both mental and physical well-being.

Manage Chronic Health Conditions

Chronic health conditions such as diabetes, hypertension, and cardiovascular disease have been associated with an increased risk of cognitive decline. Effectively managing these conditions through regular medical check-ups, medication adherence, and lifestyle modifications can contribute to preserving cognitive function.

Avoid Harmful Substances

Substance abuse, including excessive alcohol consumption and smoking, can adversely affect cognitive health. Minimizing or eliminating the use of harmful substances is a crucial step in preventing memory loss.

The Cognitive Workout: Fun and Effective Activities

Now, let us turn our attention to the enjoyable part of preventative success—the cognitive workout. Engaging in activities that are not only beneficial for the brain but also bring joy and fulfillment can make the journey toward memory preservation a delightful one.

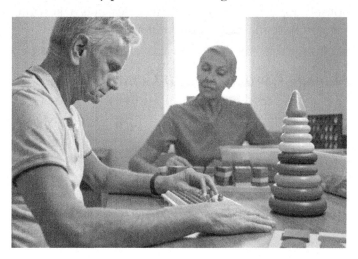

Brain Games and Puzzles

Games such as Sudoku, crossword puzzles, and memory matching not only challenge your cognitive abilities but also provide a source of entertainment. These activities stimulate different areas of the brain, enhancing memory and problem-solving skills.

Learning a New Skill

Whether it is picking up a musical instrument, learning a new language, or exploring a creative pursuit, acquiring new skills stimulates neuroplasticity—the brain's ability to adapt and form new connections. This not only enhances cognitive function but also adds richness to your life.

Cultural and Educational Activities

Attend cultural events, lectures, or workshops to feed your intellectual curiosity. Exposure to new ideas and perspectives fosters cognitive flexibility and keeps your mind active.

Physical Activities With a Cognitive Twist

Incorporate cognitive challenges into your physical activities. For example, try dancing to different types of music, practicing tai chi, or engaging in activities that require coordination and mental focus.

A Personalized Approach to Prevention

It is essential to recognize that one size does not fit all when it comes to preventative measures for memory loss. Each person is unique, with individual preferences, interests, and health considerations. Crafting a personalized approach involves exploring different strategies and finding the combination that resonates with you. Here are some tips for tailoring your approach:

- **Assess Your Lifestyle:** Reflect on your current lifestyle choices and identify areas that may benefit from improvement. Whether it is incorporating more physical activity, adjusting your diet, or prioritizing sleep, small changes can have a significant impact over time.

- **Explore Your Interests:** Choose activities that align with your interests and passions. If you enjoy music, consider learning to play an instrument. If you love nature, explore outdoor activities that combine physical exercise with the joy of being in natural surroundings.

- **Stay Consistent:** Consistency is key in preventative efforts. Establishing habits and routines that support cognitive health requires commitment and perseverance. Set realistic goals, celebrate small victories, and stay motivated on your memory-preservation journey.

- **Seek Professional Guidance:** Consult with healthcare professionals, including your primary care physician and specialists, to assess your overall health and receive personalized recommendations. They can guide managing chronic conditions, optimizing medication regimens, and addressing specific health concerns.

Realizing the Potential: Success Stories

To further underscore the potential of preventative strategies, let us explore real-life success stories of individuals who have embraced proactive measures to preserve their memory and cognitive vitality:

The Power of Lifelong Learning

Meet Margaret, a retiree who decided to learn a new language in her 70s. Engaging in regular language classes not only provided intellectual stimulation but also connected her with a vibrant community of learners. Margaret's zest for learning contributed to enhanced cognitive function and a sharper memory.

Physical Activity as a Lifestyle

John, a septuagenarian, took up daily walking as a form of exercise. What started as a simple routine evolved into a passion for hiking. Regular physical activity not only improved John's cardiovascular health but also had a positive impact on his cognitive function. Hiking became a source of joy, combining the benefits of exercise with the mental stimulation of exploring new trails.

The Social Butterfly's Secret

Susan, a retiree living alone, made a conscious effort to stay socially connected. She joined a local book club, participated in community events, and volunteered at a nearby charity. Susan's active social life not only provided emotional support but also engaged her brain in meaningful ways, contributing to cognitive resilience.

So you see, the journey to preserving and enhancing cognitive function is multifaceted, encompassing lifestyle choices, social connections, and enjoyable activities that stimulate the mind. The success stories of individuals who have embraced preventative measures underscore the transformative potential of these strategies.

As you embark on your own journey toward cognitive vitality, remember that small steps can lead to significant results. Whether you choose to incorporate brain games into your routine, explore new hobbies, or prioritize physical activity, every effort contributes to the overall health of your brain.

In Chapter 6, we will delve deeper into specific activities, games, and techniques designed to engage different aspects of memory and cognition. By embracing a holistic and personalized approach to memory preservation, you are not just preventing memory loss—you are cultivating a vibrant and fulfilling life, filled with the joy of discovery, connection, and mental agility.

Techniques for Preserving Cognitive Function

From lifestyle adjustments to engaging memory games, the following overview is a prelude to the detailed methods awaiting exploration in the next chapters of this book.

- **Lifelong Learning:** The adage "Use it or lose it" holds profound truth when it comes to cognitive health. Engaging in continuous learning, whether through formal education, workshops, or self-directed exploration, keeps the brain active and adaptable. Lifelong learning fosters the growth of new neural connections, enhancing memory and cognitive flexibility. Embrace the joy of discovery and cultivate a curious mindset to nourish your brain throughout life.

- **Physical Exercise:** The benefits of regular physical exercise extend beyond cardiovascular health—they encompass cognitive vitality as well. Exercise increases blood flow to the brain, stimulates the release of neurotransmitters, and promotes the growth of new neurons. From brisk walks to dance classes, finding enjoyable physical activities not only improves overall health but also contributes to a sharper and more resilient memory.

- **Brain-Boosting Nutrition:** A nutrient-rich diet is a cornerstone of cognitive well-being. Foods rich in antioxidants and essential vitamins support brain health and contribute to the prevention of memory loss. Incorporate colorful fruits and vegetables, whole grains, and fish into your diet. Consider consulting with a nutritionist to tailor your meals to maximize the cognitive benefits.

- **Adequate Sleep:** Quality sleep is a non-negotiable pillar of cognitive health. During sleep, the brain consolidates memories, processes information, and clears out toxins. Establishing a consistent sleep routine, creating a comfortable sleep environment, and prioritizing restful sleep are crucial components of preventing memory loss.

- **Stress Management:** Chronic stress has been linked to cognitive decline, making stress management an integral part of preventative measures. Practices such as meditation, deep breathing exercises, and mindfulness not only alleviate stress but also support cognitive resilience. Embrace relaxation techniques to nurture both your mental and emotional well-being.

- **Social Engagement:** Human connections play a pivotal role in cognitive health. Maintaining strong social ties contributes to emotional well-being and provides opportunities for intellectual stimulation. Participate in social activities, join clubs, or volunteer to foster a sense of connection and purpose. Social engagement is not only enjoyable but also a potent ally in preventing memory loss.

- **Cognitive Challenges:** Just as physical exercise strengthens the body, cognitive challenges fortify the mind. Engage in activities that require mental effort, such as puzzles, games, and learning new skills. These activities stimulate various regions of the brain, enhancing memory, attention, and problem-solving abilities. Explore the vast array of memory games and cognitive exercises designed to keep your mind agile and vibrant.

- **Regular Health Checkups:** Monitoring and managing overall health is a fundamental aspect of preventing memory loss. Regular checkups with healthcare professionals can help identify and address potential risk factors, such as high blood pressure, diabetes, or other medical conditions that may impact cognitive function. Stay proactive in managing your health to safeguard your brain.

- **Balancing Work and Leisure:** Achieving a balance between work and leisure is crucial for cognitive well-being. Chronic overwork and stress can contribute to cognitive decline. Finding a harmonious balance between responsibilities and leisure pursuits fosters a healthier and more resilient mind.

- **Mindfulness Practices:** Mindfulness practices, such as meditation and yoga, cultivate a heightened awareness of the present moment. These practices have been associated with improvements in attention, memory, and overall cognitive function. Integrate mindfulness into your daily routine to enhance mental clarity and promote a positive mindset.

- **Stay Hydrated:** Proper hydration is often overlooked but plays a vital role in cognitive function. Dehydration can impair concentration and memory. Ensure you maintain adequate fluid intake throughout the day to support optimal brain function.

- **Stay Mentally Active:** Challenging your brain with diverse mental activities is a potent strategy for preventing memory loss. Reading, writing, engaging in intellectual discussions, and pursuing hobbies that require mental effort contribute to cognitive vitality. Keep your mind active and adaptable by introducing variety into your mental pursuits.

- **Manage Medications:** If you are on medication, it is crucial to manage and monitor your medication regimen. Some medications may impact cognitive function as a side effect. Regularly consult with your healthcare provider to ensure that your medications are optimized for both your physical and cognitive well-being.

- **Limit Alcohol and Avoid Smoking:** Excessive alcohol consumption and smoking have been linked to cognitive decline (Jjavaid, 2024). Limiting alcohol intake and avoiding smoking are essential steps in preserving cognitive health.

These lifestyle choices contribute not only to overall well-being but also to a sharper and more resilient memory.

This overview serves as a foundational guide, providing a comprehensive blueprint for preventing memory loss. Remember that the key to success lies in personalization—tailoring these strategies to align with your preferences, interests, and individual needs.

Embark on this journey with a spirit of curiosity and commitment. By integrating these proven methods into your life, you are not just preventing memory loss—you are actively cultivating a resilient and vibrant cognitive landscape. Your brain is a remarkable organ capable of adaptation and growth, and with the right tools and mindset, you can enhance your cognitive capacity and enjoy a life filled with mental acuity, joy, and fulfillment.

In this chapter, we have journeyed through the landscape of memory loss prevalence, dispelling misconceptions and unveiling the multifaceted nature of cognitive health. The key takeaways include understanding the various stages of memory loss, the impact on different parts of the brain, and most importantly, the empowering realization that prevention is not only possible but within reach.

This chapter lays the foundation for the broader framework of our quest to enhance cognitive and memory capacity. It underscores the significance of proactive measures, lifestyle choices, and engaging activities in maintaining a resilient and vibrant memory.

As we move to the next chapter, the focus sharpens on the delightful realm of "preventative fun"—a collection of enjoyable activities and games specifically designed to fortify your memory and invigorate your cognitive prowess. Get ready to infuse your journey with joy and excitement, as we explore the power of play in the pursuit of cognitive well-being.

Chapter 3:

Preventative Fun

Memory is the sense of loss, and loss pulls us after it. –
Marilynne Robinson

Welcome to the vibrant world of preventative fun, where we embark on a journey to fortify the fortress of our minds against the passage of time. This chapter is dedicated to empowering you with proven strategies, engaging activities, and delightful games that not only stave off memory loss but also infuse your life with joy and mental resilience.

In the pages ahead, we will explore strategies and methods carefully curated to enhance your cognitive capacities. Forget the notion that memory decline is an inevitable part of aging; instead, embrace the exciting prospect of actively participating in the preservation of your mental acuity. These strategies are not just tools; they are gateways to a more fulfilling and vibrant life.

As you immerse yourself in the following pages, you will discover that preventing memory loss can be a joyful and entertaining endeavor. From stimulating brain exercises to immersive games that tickle your neurons, each recommendation is rooted in scientific research and designed to transform the quest for memory enhancement into an enjoyable adventure.

By the time you reach the end of this chapter, you will not only have a collection of proven techniques at your disposal but also a renewed confidence in your ability to safeguard your cognitive well-being.

Memory Loss Games: Sharpening the Mind With Play

Let us start with the captivating realm of memory loss games—entertaining activities designed not only to bring joy to your leisure hours but also to fortify the cognitive fortresses that safeguard your memory.

Sudoku, Rebus Puzzles, and Chess

Sudoku: A Symphony of Numbers

Sudoku is a classic number puzzle game that originated in Japan. The game consists of a 9x9 grid, divided into nine 3x3 subgrids. The objective is to fill in the grid with numbers from 1 to 9, ensuring that each row, each column, and each 3x3 subgrid contains all of the numbers without repetition.

1	3			5	4	9		
			7			6	5	
6			2	1	9			
	2	9			7			
	4		1				3	2
5	6			4				7
							7	
4	7					6		

Getting Started

- **Learn the Basics:** Familiarize yourself with the rules of Sudoku. Understand how to fill in the grid while adhering to the constraints of no repetition in rows, columns, and subgrids.

- **Start Simple:** Begin with easy puzzles and gradually progress to more challenging ones as you gain confidence. Many newspapers and online platforms offer Sudoku puzzles of varying difficulty levels.

- **Practice Regularly:** Consistency is key. Dedicate a specific time each day to tackle a Sudoku puzzle. The more you practice, the more comfortable and adept you become.

How It Improves Memory

- **Enhances Logical Thinking:** Sudoku requires logical deduction and problem-solving skills. Engaging in such mental exercises regularly helps strengthen neural connections associated with logical reasoning.

- **Improves Concentration:** The game demands sustained attention as you analyze and assess potential number placements. This focused concentration can translate into improved overall cognitive function, including memory.

- **Memory Recall:** Remembering the numbers already placed in the grid and recalling potential placements exercise short-term memory, contributing to its sharpening over time.

Where to Find Sudokus

- Puzzle Society

- DailyCaring

- Puzzles.ca

Rebus Puzzles: Unraveling Visual Conundrums

According to Mental Bomb (2024), "A Rebus puzzle is a form of word puzzle that uses pictures or symbols to represent words or parts of words." It challenges you to decipher a hidden message or phrase by interpreting the visual cues presented.

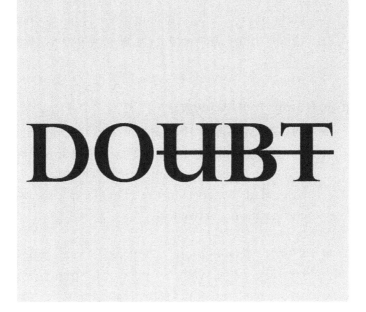

Getting Started

- **Understand the Symbols:** Familiarize yourself with common symbols used in Rebus puzzles, such as pictures, letters, and numbers that represent words or sounds.

- **Start With Easy Puzzles:** Begin with simpler Rebus puzzles and gradually progress to more intricate ones. Online platforms and puzzle books are great resources for a variety of difficulty levels.

- **Think Creatively:** Embrace a creative mindset. Rebus puzzles often require thinking outside the box and making unconventional connections between visual elements and language.

How It Improves Memory

- **Visual Memory Enhancement:** Deciphering the visual symbols in Rebus puzzles stimulates and enhances visual memory. This can be particularly beneficial for recalling faces, objects, and details in everyday life.

- **Word Association:** Making connections between visual symbols and words strengthens associative memory. This can improve the brain's ability to recall related information and enhance verbal memory skills.

- **Cognitive Flexibility:** Rebus puzzles encourage thinking from multiple perspectives, fostering cognitive flexibility. This mental agility can contribute to better memory retention and retrieval.

Where to Find Rebus Puzzles

- Scholastic

- ESL Vault

- Reader's Digest

Chess: A Strategic Mind Workout

Chess is a timeless strategic board game that engages two players in a battle of wits. Each player commands an army of distinct pieces with unique movements, aiming to checkmate their opponent's king.

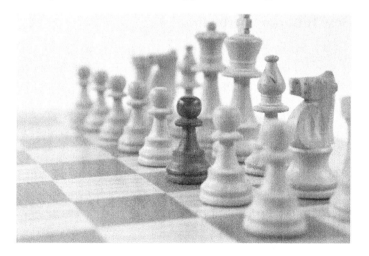

Getting Started

- **Learn the Rules:** Understand the movements and rules associated with each Chess piece.

Mastering the basics is crucial for enjoying the strategic depth of the game.

- **Play Regularly:** Engage in regular Chess matches, whether against a friend, a computer opponent or through online platforms. Practice is essential for honing your strategic thinking skills.

- **Study Strategies:** Explore different Chess strategies and tactics. Books, online tutorials, and Chess Clubs are excellent resources for expanding your Chess repertoire.

How It Improves Memory

- **Strategic Thinking:** Chess is a game of strategy and foresight. Planning moves in advance and anticipating your opponent's responses stimulate strategic thinking, which can enhance memory by reinforcing planning and organization skills.

- **Pattern Recognition:** Recognizing and remembering common Chess patterns, such as openings and tactics, exercises pattern recognition abilities. This skill can be transferred to everyday life, aiding in memory recall of familiar sequences.

- **Working Memory:** Chess involves holding multiple pieces of information in your mind simultaneously, exercising your working memory. As this mental muscle strengthens, so does your ability to process and recall information efficiently.

Where to Play Chess

- Chess.com

- Chess Arena

- Poki

Memory loss games are not just pastimes; they are powerful tools for fortifying your cognitive abilities. Sudoku, Rebus puzzles, and Chess each offer a unique set of challenges that stimulate various aspects of memory and cognitive function. Remember that the joy of play is intertwined with the enhancement of your mental prowess. So, let the challenges excite you, and witness the magic as your memory becomes more resilient, agile, and ready for the adventures that lie ahead.

Memory Matching Cards: A Visual Symphony for the Mind

Creating Your Memory Matching Cards

Memory matching cards are engaging games designed to stimulate your memory while providing hours of entertainment. The beauty of this activity lies in its simplicity and adaptability. Whether you choose to use pictures, words, colors, or a combination, the goal remains the same: to match pairs and exercise your memory muscles.

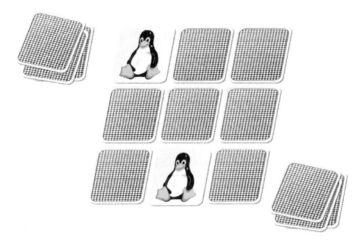

Materials Needed

- Cardstock or thick paper for creating sturdy cards

- Markers, colored pencils, or stickers to add visual elements to your cards

- Scissors for cutting out the cards

- Storage container to keep your cards organized

Instructions

Step 1: Design Your Cards

- **Choose a Theme:** Decide on the theme of your memory matching cards. It could be anything from animals and nature to famous landmarks or even family photos. The key is to make it enjoyable and personally meaningful.

- **Create Pairs:** For each card, make an identical twin. If you are using pictures, ensure you have two copies of each image. If words or colors are your preference, ensure each pair is identical.

- **Add Visual Appeal:** Use markers, colored pencils, or stickers to enhance the visual appeal of your cards. Bright colors and clear images will make the game more engaging.

Step 2: Print or Copy Your Cards

- **Print Option:** If you have access to a printer, design your cards digitally using software or an online tool, and print them on cardstock for durability.

- **Handmade Option:** If you prefer a hands-on approach, draw, color, or paste images directly onto the cardstock. Cut them out carefully to ensure neat and uniform cards.

Step 3: Set Up the Game

- **Shuffle the Deck:** Once you have your set of memory matching cards, shuffle them well. This step ensures that the cards are in a random order each time you play.

- **Layout the Cards:** Place the cards face down in a grid formation. The size of the grid can vary based on the number of cards you have and the level of difficulty you desire.

Step 4: Playing the Game

- **Take Turns:** The game is typically played with one or more players. Players take turns flipping over two cards at a time, to find matching pairs.

- **Remember and Match:** As cards are turned over, memorize the placement and content of each card. The objective is to match pairs by recalling the location of identical cards.

- **Continue Until All Pairs Are Found:** The game continues until all pairs are successfully matched. The winner is the player with the most matches.

Step 5: Variations and Challenges

- **Increase Difficulty:** As you become more adept, increase the challenge by adding more cards to the grid or by reducing the time allowed for each turn.

- **Theme Switch:** Switch themes periodically to keep the game fresh and provide a varied stimulus for your memory.

Benefits of Memory Matching Cards

- **Memory Enhancement:** The game exercises your short-term memory as you strive to remember the location and content of each card.

- **Focus and Concentration:** Playing memory matching cards requires concentration and attention, contributing to improved focus.

- **Pattern Recognition:** Matching identical pairs hones your pattern recognition skills, which can extend to various aspects of daily life.

If You Want to Play Matching Cards Online

- <u>Lumosity</u>

- <u>Memozor</u>

- <u>Interacty</u>

So you see, memory matching cards are a dynamic workout for your mind. The creative process of designing your cards and the mental challenge of matching pairs combine to create an activity that is both enjoyable and beneficial for cognitive health. So, gather your materials, unleash your creativity, and let the matching games begin! As you engage in this preventative fun, revel in the joy of play while knowing that you are actively nurturing and preserving the vibrant landscape of your memory.

License Plate Memory Game: Unveiling the Memory Matrix on the Road

Did you know that the very act of driving can be transformed into a fun and effective memory-enhancing activity? Many people use the familiar sight of license plates as an opportunity to engage their minds and keep their memory sharp. In this activity, we will explore how you can turn your daily commute or leisurely drives into a captivating license plate memory game.

Game 1: Memory Challenge - The Number Crunch

How to Play

- **Select a Time Frame:** Decide on a specific time duration for the game, such as the duration of your commute or a set period during a road trip.

- **Observation Mode:** As you drive, pay close attention to the license plates of the vehicles around you. Focus on memorizing the numbers and letters on each plate.

- **Memory Recall:** After the designated time frame, challenge yourself to recall as many license plate numbers as possible. Try to remember both the numbers and the sequence of letters accurately.

- **Scoring:** Keep a mental or written tally of the plates you successfully recall. Award yourself points for each accurate match.

- **Level Up:** Gradually increase the difficulty by extending the time frame or by challenging yourself to remember more plates in each session.

Benefits

- **Visual Memory Enhancement:** The game exercises your visual memory as you actively observe and memorize license plate details.

- **Concentration Boost:** Maintaining focus on the road while simultaneously engaging in a memory challenge sharpens your concentration skills.

- **Memory Retention:** Regular play enhances your ability to retain and recall information, contributing to overall memory improvement.

Game 2: Wordplay Challenge - License Plate Lingo

How to Play

- **Word Formation:** Instead of memorizing the entire license plate, focus on creating words or phrases using the letters on a plate.

- **Unleash Creativity:** Rearrange the letters to form as many words as possible. Challenge yourself to create longer and more complex words.

- **Themed Rounds:** Introduce themes for word creation, such as animals, colors, or places. This adds an extra layer of creativity and mental stimulation.

- **Share and Compare:** If you have a driving companion, take turns sharing the words you formed. Compare your creations and appreciate the diverse interpretations.

Benefits

- **Language Skills:** License Plate Lingo stimulates your creativity and language skills as you craft words from seemingly random combinations of letters.

- **Flexibility of Thought:** The game encourages flexible thinking, fostering cognitive adaptability and the ability to see multiple possibilities.

- **Social Interaction:** If you are driving with others, the game becomes a delightful way to engage in friendly competition and share a few laughs.

This memory game is a testament to the potential for cognitive enhancement in the most unexpected places.

Transforming the mundane task of observing license plates into a memory challenge not only makes your drives more enjoyable but also actively contributes to the maintenance and improvement of your cognitive functions.

Improving Brain Productivity: Connecting the Dots for Cognitive Resilience

The mind thrives on stimulation and engagement, and here, we explore how activities like reading, learning an instrument, practicing math, and journaling can serve as powerful tools to keep the brain sharp. Let us delve into each activity and uncover the secrets to boosting brain productivity.

Reading: Nourishing the Mind With Words

How Reading Makes Connections

Reading regularly creates new neural pathways in the brain, fostering connections between different regions. As you immerse yourself in a book, your brain forms associations between characters, plotlines, and settings.

It also is a cognitive workout. It engages various brain regions, including those responsible for language processing, imagination, and empathy. The act of decoding words and comprehending their meanings strengthens the brain's cognitive capabilities.

Reading exposes you to a multitude of perspectives and ideas, encouraging your brain to make connections between your existing knowledge and new information. This process enhances critical thinking and expands your mental horizons.

Tips for Reading

- **Diversify Your Reading List:** Explore various genres, from fiction and non-fiction to poetry and memoirs. Diversifying your reading material exposes your brain to different writing styles and subjects.

- **Discuss What You Read:** Engage in book clubs and discussions, or simply share your thoughts with a friend. Explaining your understanding of a book helps reinforce the connections your brain made during the reading process.

- **Set Reading Goals:** Challenge yourself to read a certain number of books within a specific time frame. Setting goals not only keeps you motivated but also ensures a continuous flow of mental stimulation.

Learn an Instrument: A Symphony for Cognitive Harmony

How Learning an Instrument Makes Connections

Playing a musical instrument requires the coordination of multiple tasks, such as reading sheet music, controlling your breath, and manipulating the instrument itself. This multitasking enhances the connections between different areas of the brain.

Learning and memorizing musical pieces stimulate the memory centers of the brain. As you commit notes, rhythms, and techniques to memory, you are actively strengthening your cognitive recall abilities.

Music has a profound emotional impact. Learning to express yourself through an instrument fosters connections between your emotions and your creative outlets, promoting emotional intelligence and well-being.

Tips for Learning an Instrument

- **Start Small:** Begin with a relatively easy instrument if you are a beginner. As you gradually build proficiency, you can explore more complex instruments.

- **Consistent Practice:** Regular and consistent practice is key to making progress. Set aside dedicated time each day to practice, even if it is just for a short duration.

- **Take Lessons:** Consider taking lessons from a professional or using online resources. Structured learning environments provide guidance and help accelerate your progress.

Practice Math: Exercising the Brain's Logical Muscles

How Practicing Math Makes Connections

Math is inherently logical, requiring the brain to follow step-by-step processes to arrive at solutions. Engaging in math exercises enhances your logical reasoning skills, making connections between problems and solutions.

Math problems present unique challenges that require creative problem-solving. By practicing math regularly, you train your brain to approach problems from different angles, strengthening your problem-solving capabilities.

Math involves memorizing formulas, concepts, and patterns. Practicing math regularly improves your memory and enhances your ability to maintain focus, critical for overall cognitive health.

Tips for Practicing Math

- **Start at Your Comfort Level:** Begin with math problems that match your current skill level. As you gain confidence, gradually progress to more challenging exercises.

- **Real-Life Application:** Connect math to real-life situations. Whether it is budgeting, measuring ingredients for a recipe, or calculating travel distances, applying math in practical ways reinforces its relevance.

- **Consistency Is Key:** Dedicate a specific time each day or week to practice math. Consistent practice builds a strong foundation and keeps your mathematical skills sharp.

Journaling: Unleashing the Power of Reflection

How Journaling Makes Connections

Journaling encourages introspection and self-reflection. By putting thoughts on paper, you create connections between your experiences, emotions, and perceptions, leading to a deeper understanding of yourself and the world around you.

Writing about your emotions and experiences fosters emotional intelligence. As you articulate your feelings, your brain establishes connections between emotions and language, promoting emotional awareness and regulation.

Journaling about your day or significant events helps consolidate memories. The act of putting pen to paper strengthens the neural pathways associated with the events you are recording.

Journal Prompts

- **Daily Gratitude:** Write about three things you are grateful for each day. This practice helps your brain focus on positive aspects, promoting a positive outlook on life.

- **Reflect on Challenges:** Journal about a recent challenge or obstacle you faced and how you overcame it. This reflection encourages problem-solving skills and resilience.

- **Dream Journaling:** Record your dreams in the morning. This not only engages your creative mind but also aids in the recall of dream content, exercising your memory.

- **Future Self Reflection:** Describe the person you aspire to be in the future. Reflect on the steps you can take to align your actions with your vision.

Engaging in activities that foster connections and stimulate various cognitive functions is key to maintaining mental sharpness. Whether you choose to lose yourself in the pages of a book or pour your thoughts onto paper through journaling, each activity contributes uniquely to the cognitive symphony playing in your brain. Embrace the diversity of these activities, make them a part of your routine, and witness the profound impact they can have on your cognitive well-being.

In this chapter on preventative fun, we discovered the transformative power of engaging in activities like reading, learning an instrument, practicing math, and journaling. These enjoyable pursuits not only fostered connections in our brains but also laid the foundation for cognitive resilience. As we traverse the world of preventative fun, we have come to appreciate that keeping our minds sharp is not only about exercise and challenges but also about relishing the joy inherent in these activities.

This chapter holds an important role in the broader framework of our memory improvement journey. By integrating these diverse and enjoyable activities into our routines, we fortify the foundation upon which memory enhancement strategies can flourish. The combination of preventative fun and targeted strategies creates a holistic approach to maintaining cognitive health, unlocking the full potential of our minds.

As we look forward, the next chapter will unveil a treasure trove of memory improvement strategies. From mnemonic devices to mindfulness techniques, we will delve into practical methods that empower you to enhance memory and cognitive function. Get ready to embark on a focused exploration of the strategies that will shape your memory's future.

Chapter 4:

Memory Improvement Strategies

There are memories that time does not erase... Forever does not make loss forgettable, only bearable. –Cassandra Clare

Let us move to the preservation and enhancement of one of our most precious assets—our memory. As we navigate the golden years of life, it is only natural to become more conscious of our cognitive abilities and the potential changes that may occur. Fear not, for this chapter is designed to be your guide, your companion on a journey toward boosting and safeguarding your memory.

In the realm of memory improvement, the key is proactive engagement. We are here to unveil a trove of enjoyable and proven activities that not only serve as a shield against memory decline but also add a spark of joy to your daily routine. Whether you are concerned about potential memory loss or simply want to stay sharp and agile, the strategies and activities within these pages are tailored just for you.

While it primarily serves as a preventative measure, those facing more significant memory challenges can find solace and practical solutions within these lines. We believe in the power of resilience and the human capacity for growth, no matter the stage of life.

So, through engaging games, stimulating exercises, and enjoyable activities, we will not only sharpen our minds but also cultivate a sense of joy in the process. The journey to memory enhancement is an adventure, and you are about to set sail with a compass filled with proven techniques, wisdom, and, most importantly, the joy of learning.

Game: Memory Mastery Match-Up

The memory mastery match-up is a delightful card game designed to not only entertain but also enhance cognitive functions, including memory. It combines elements of strategy, attention, and a touch of luck to make for an engaging experience. This game is perfect for socializing with friends or family while subtly exercising your memory muscles.

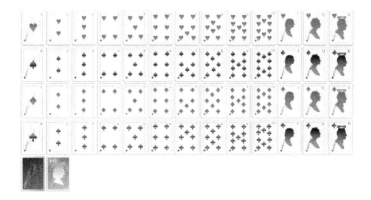

Materials

- A standard deck of playing cards

Instructions

- Use a standard 52-card deck

- Shuffle the cards thoroughly

Card Distribution

- Deal each player an equal number of cards, face-down.

- The number of cards per player depends on the total number of players, ensuring an equal distribution.

Gameplay

- Players take turns laying down a card from their hand in the center, forming a communal pile.

- The goal is to create pairs of cards with matching ranks (numbers or faces).

- For example, if a player places a 7 of hearts, the next player can lay down another 7 (from a different suit) to create a pair.

- When a pair is formed, those cards are set aside, and the player gets another turn.

Memory Challenge
- To add a memory-enhancing element, players must briefly memorize the cards laid in the communal pile.

- If a player hesitates or fails to remember the cards correctly, they may draw a penalty card (face-down) from the deck.

- Penalty cards act as negative points at the end of the game.

Winning the Game
- The game continues until all pairs are formed and no more cards remain in the players' hands.

- The player with the most pairs wins.

- To declare the overall winner, subtract any penalty cards from their total pairs.

Optional Variations

- For an added challenge, introduce a time limit for memorization.

- Create custom rules for special cards (e.g., skip a turn, reverse direction) to keep the game dynamic.

- Remember, the primary focus is on enjoying the game, but the subtle memory challenges incorporated into this game make it an excellent tool for cognitive enhancement.

Game: Word Workout

Crossword Connection

Engage your mind in a crossword puzzle that not only tests your vocabulary but also challenges your memory recall.

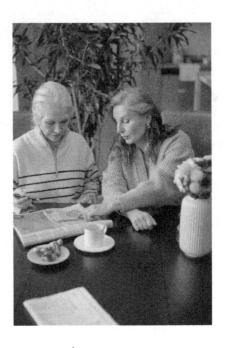

Materials Needed

- A crossword puzzle from a newspaper, magazine, or online source

- A pen or pencil

Instructions

- Start by selecting a crossword puzzle that matches your skill level.

- Begin solving the puzzle by filling in the words you know.

- As you encounter more challenging clues, take a moment to recall related words or associations from your memory.

- Work on the puzzle gradually, allowing breaks if needed, and return to it with fresh eyes.

- The process of remembering words and making connections boosts your memory capabilities.

If You Want to Play Crosswords Online
- Arkadium

- Puzzle Society

- The Guardian

Word Search Wanderlust

Embark on a word search adventure that not only entertains but also strengthens your attention to detail and pattern recognition.

Materials Needed
- Word search puzzle from a book or online source

- A pen or pencil

Instructions

- Select a word search puzzle with words relevant to your interests.

- Carefully scan the grid for the hidden words.

- As you find each word, take a moment to reflect on its meaning or use it in a sentence.

- Focus on the process of locating words and recalling their definitions, enhancing both short-term and long-term memory.

- Enjoy the visual aspect of recognizing patterns and connections within the grid.

Word Search Puzzles Online

RedWood RedWordle

Arkadium

Poki

Memory Lane Anagrams

Exercise your brain with anagram challenges, promoting quick thinking, language skills, and memory recall.

Materials Needed

- List of mixed-up words (anagrams) on a sheet of paper or generated using an online tool

- A pen or pencil

Instructions

- Obtain a list of anagrams or create your own by scrambling the letters of common words.

- Unscramble each word, keeping track of the time it takes to solve them.

- Reflect on the words as you unravel them, reinforcing your memory of spelling and word structures.

- Challenge yourself with more complex anagrams over time, gradually enhancing your memory and cognitive flexibility.

- Share the activity with friends or family for a friendly competition, making it a social and memory-boosting experience.

Anagrams Online

Pogo

Writing Exercises

Remember, the goal is not just to solve the puzzles but to engage your brain actively. These word puzzles serve as enjoyable tools to maintain and enhance cognitive function while providing a sense of accomplishment and joy. So, dive into the world of words and let the memory workout begin!

Mindful Memory Meditation

Meditation, often associated with relaxation and stress reduction, is a powerful tool that can significantly contribute to memory improvement. By fostering a calm and focused mind, meditation helps reduce cognitive overload, enhances attention, and supports the consolidation of memories.

Guided Meditation Scripts

Focused Breath Meditation for Clarity

1. Sit comfortably in a quiet space.

2. Gently close your eyes and take a few deep breaths, inhaling through your nose and exhaling through your mouth.

3. Direct your attention to your breath. Feel the sensation of each inhale and exhale.

4. As you breathe, imagine inhaling a calming energy that clears your mind and exhaling any tension or clutter.

5. Now, shift your focus to a specific memory you would like to enhance. Visualize the details, colors, and emotions associated with that memory.

6. With each breath, allow the memory to become clearer and more vivid. If distractions arise, acknowledge them gently and bring your focus back to the memory.

7. Continue this practice for 5-10 minutes, gradually bringing awareness back to your surroundings as you conclude.

Body Scan Meditation for Memory Recall

1. Lie down or sit comfortably, ensuring your spine is straight. Close your eyes.

2. Begin by bringing attention to your toes. Feel any sensations or tension, then consciously release it as you exhale.

3. Slowly move your awareness up through each part of your body, releasing tension and promoting relaxation.

4. As you reach your head, focus on the area where memories are stored. Picture a soft light illuminating this region, symbolizing clarity and access to memories.

5. Allow your mind to wander to a specific memory you want to recall. Engage your senses in this visualization, immersing yourself in the details.

6. If the memory is elusive, be patient. Sometimes, simply creating a calm mental space can encourage memories to surface.

7. Spend 10-15 minutes in this body scan, concluding with a few deep breaths before returning to your day.

Loving-Kindness Meditation for Positive Associations

1. Sit comfortably, close your eyes, and take a few deep breaths to center yourself.

2. Begin by sending feelings of love and kindness to yourself. Visualize a warm, radiant light surrounding you, fostering a sense of self-compassion.

3. Extend these feelings to someone you care about, picturing them surrounded by the same warm light.

4. Gradually, broaden your focus to include friends, family, and even acquaintances. Wish them well, imagining their happiness and fulfillment.

5. As you cultivate positive emotions, think of a memory associated with joy and connection. Allow this memory to unfold in your mind, savoring the positive emotions.

6. Continue this meditation for 10-15 minutes, ending with a few moments of gratitude for the memories and connections in your life.

These guided meditations offer a holistic approach to memory enhancement by promoting mental clarity, relaxation, and positive associations. Incorporate them into your routine regularly to experience the cumulative benefits of a mindful memory practice.

Game: Mindful Memory Bingo

Mindfulness is a powerful tool that can significantly contribute to improving memory and cognitive function. By engaging in mindfulness activities, individuals can enhance their focus, attention, and overall mental well-being. Mindfulness involves being fully present and aware of the current moment. When we practice mindfulness, we cultivate a heightened sense of attention and concentration. This focused awareness can directly impact memory by reducing cognitive distractions and promoting better retention of information. By incorporating mindfulness into your daily life, you create an environment conducive to optimal cognitive function and memory recall.

Now, we will explore the connection between mindfulness and memory, and we will introduce a fun and interactive way for you to incorporate mindfulness into your daily routine—mindful memory bingo.

Mindful Memory Bingo

Below is a bingo board with nine different mindfulness activities. Your goal is to engage in these activities daily and mark off each square as you complete them. Aim for a "Bingo" every day to reap the cumulative benefits of mindfulness on your memory and overall well-being.

Mindful Memory Bingo Board

Deep breathing exercise	Mindful walking	Body scan meditation
Mindful eating	Gratitude journaling	Sensory awareness
Guided meditation	Mindful listening	Digital detox

How to Play
- Complete each mindfulness activity daily.

- Mark off the corresponding square on your bingo board for each completed activity.

- Aim for a full row (horizontal, vertical, or diagonal) or fill the entire board to achieve "Bingo."

By incorporating these mindfulness activities into your daily routine, you not only work toward enhancing your memory but also promote overall mental clarity and well-being. So, let the mindfulness journey begin, and may you hit "Bingo" daily!

The Pursuit of New Skills

In the quest for a sharper memory and a more resilient cognitive function, one of the most effective strategies is to embrace the pursuit of new skills. Learning engages our brains, fosters neuroplasticity, and creates new neural connections, all of which contribute to improved memory. Below is a list of diverse skills, each accompanied by an explanation of how it can benefit and enhance your memory.

1. **Learning a Musical Instrument:** Enhances auditory memory and motor coordination.

2. **Mastering a New Language:** Boosts cognitive flexibility and strengthens memory recall.

3. **Trying Photography:** Sharpens visual memory and attention to detail.

4. **Exploring Painting or Drawing:** Enhances creativity and improves spatial memory.

5. **Practicing Yoga or Meditation:** Reduces stress, leading to improved overall cognitive function.

6. **Cooking or Baking:** Strengthens procedural memory.

7. **Gardening:** Boosts memory through the nurturing of plants and the environment.

8. **Knitting or Crocheting:** Improves focus and fine motor skills, benefiting memory.

9. **Coding or Programming:** Enhances problem-solving abilities and logical thinking.

10. **Chess or Strategic Board Games:** Sharpens strategic planning and spatial memory.

11. **Dancing:** Combines physical activity with rhythm, benefiting memory.

12. **Joining a Book Club:** Expands vocabulary and fosters narrative memory.

13. **Learning Calligraphy:** Enhances fine motor skills and attention to detail.

14. **Mindful Walking:** Improves spatial awareness and overall attention.

15. **Bird Watching**: Enhances observation skills and memory for species details.

16. **Volunteering:** Fosters a sense of purpose, improving overall cognitive health.

17. **Playing Memory Games:** Engages directly with memory functions for a targeted boost.

18. **Taking Up Astronomy:** Stimulates curiosity and improves attention to celestial details.

19. **Studying Art History:** Enhances visual memory and cultural awareness.

20. **Learning a New Dance Style:** Combines physical exercise with memory for choreography.

21. **Blogging or Journaling:** Improves verbal memory and self-reflection.

22. **Mindful Coloring:** Promotes relaxation and improves focus.

23. **Playing a New Sport:** Combines physical activity with strategic thinking.

24. **Mastering Origami:** Enhances spatial reasoning and fine motor skills.

25. **Practicing Mindful Breathing:** Improves focus and reduces stress, benefiting memory.

26. **Learning Basic Sign Language:** Strengthens visual memory and communication skills.

27. **Studying Philosophy:** Stimulates critical thinking and logical memory.

28. **Creative Writing:** Enhances verbal memory and creativity.

29. **Sudoku or Crossword Puzzles:** Boosts problem-solving skills and memory recall.

30. **DIY Home Repairs:** Engages problem-solving abilities and procedural memory.

Each of these skills offers a unique pathway to stimulating your brain and enhancing your memory. Choose the ones that resonate with you, and enjoy the journey of discovery and cognitive empowerment.

In this chapter, we explored engaging activities, from memory-boosting games to mindfulness practices and the acquisition of new skills, all designed to fortify and enhance cognitive function. These strategies not only offer enjoyment but serve as potent tools in our quest to preserve and sharpen memory.

Looking ahead, our journey continues into the realm of understanding severe memory loss. The next chapter delves into compassion, knowledge, and practical insights for individuals navigating the complexities of profound memory challenges. Join me as we explore the nuances of memory loss, providing support and guidance for those on this unique and often challenging path.

Chapter 5:

Understanding Severe Memory Loss

Memories and thoughts age, just as people do. But certain thoughts can never age, and certain memories can never fade. –
Haruki Murakami

Whether you find yourself occasionally misplacing keys or facing more profound memory lapses, this chapter is crafted with empathy and knowledge to guide you through the labyrinth of severe memory loss. It is not a solitary journey; countless individuals share similar concerns, and through this exploration, you will gain insights that will illuminate the path ahead.

This newfound understanding will lay a solid foundation, preparing you for the constructive steps and engaging activities we will explore together in the subsequent chapter. So, let us begin this journey of self-awareness and discovery, acknowledging memory's nuances and unveiling the potential for growth that lies within.

Severe Memory Loss

As it was mentioned in previous chapters, memory is a complex thing that unifies our experiences, thoughts, and emotions. As we age, it is natural to encounter occasional forgetfulness or minor lapses in memory. Misplacing keys, forgetting names momentarily, or blanking on a specific detail are common occurrences, often regarded as part of the normal aging process. However, within this spectrum of memory challenges, there exists a distinct category that demands special attention and understanding—severe memory loss.

Severe memory loss transcends the realm of occasional forgetfulness. It is characterized by a significant and persistent decline in cognitive function, impacting daily life and hindering the ability to perform routine tasks. Distinguishing severe memory loss from more benign forms is crucial for seniors to comprehend the nature of their cognitive challenges.

Normal memory issues might involve occasional forgetfulness or the inability to recall details swiftly, but they do not substantially disrupt daily life. Severe memory loss, on the other hand, manifests as a profound struggle to remember critical information, such as names of close family members, important dates, or even the ability to recognize familiar surroundings.

As we delve into the depths of it, remember that knowledge is a powerful ally. By comprehending the specific challenges posed by severe memory loss, you are better positioned to explore strategies and activities that can contribute to cognitive well-being and enhance the quality of life.

Signs and Impact of Severe Memory Loss

Recognizing the signs and impact of severe memory loss is a crucial step in understanding this complex cognitive challenge. By familiarizing yourself with these indicators, you gain insight into the nuances of this condition and can take proactive measures to address its effects. Let us delve into the signs and impact of severe memory loss.

Persistent Forgetfulness

- **Sign:** Forgetting crucial information regularly, such as appointments, important dates, or names of close family members and friends.

- **Impact:** Disruption of daily life and potential strain on personal relationships due to the consistent inability to recall essential details.

Difficulty in Learning and Retaining New Information

- **Sign:** Struggling to grasp and remember new information, experiences, or skills.

- **Impact:** Impaired ability to acquire new knowledge and skills, hindering adaptability and learning in various aspects of life.

Confusion With Time and Place

- **Sign:** Losing track of time and dates, or being disoriented about one's location.

- **Impact:** Difficulty in maintaining a consistent daily routine, potential safety concerns, and challenges in organizing and planning activities.

Repetition of Questions or Statements

- **Sign:** Frequently asking the same questions or making repetitive statements within a short timeframe.

- **Impact:** Communication challenges and potential frustration for both the individual experiencing memory loss and those around them.

Misplacing Items

- **Sign:** Regularly misplacing personal belongings or putting them in unusual locations.

- **Impact:** Disorganization, frustration, and the need for assistance to locate everyday items, contributing to a sense of dependency.

Difficulty in Problem-Solving

- **Sign:** Struggling to make decisions or solve problems, even those previously handled with ease.

- **Impact:** Impaired ability to manage daily tasks, potentially leading to heightened stress and a diminished sense of control.

Mood and Personality Changes

- **Sign:** Shifts in mood, behavior, or personality that are not consistent with the individual's usual traits.

- **Impact:** Strain on relationships, potential withdrawal from social activities, and challenges in maintaining emotional well-being.

The effects of severe memory loss extend beyond mere forgetfulness; they intricately weave into the fabric of daily life, influencing various aspects of an individual's well-being. Recognizing these impacts is fundamental in comprehending the challenges faced by seniors dealing with severe memory loss.

One profound impact is the strain on interpersonal relationships. Persistent forgetfulness and the inability to recall names or shared experiences may lead to frustration and confusion, both for the individual experiencing memory loss and their loved ones. Communication gaps may widen, and the shared history that forms the foundation of relationships may become fragmented.

In addition, severe memory loss can disrupt the individual's daily routine and ability to carry out essential tasks. The challenges in remembering appointments, managing medications, or organizing activities may contribute to feelings of helplessness and dependency. This impact not only affects the individual's sense of autonomy but also poses practical challenges in maintaining a quality lifestyle.

Furthermore, the emotional toll of severe memory loss should not be underestimated. Individuals grappling with memory loss may experience heightened levels of stress, anxiety, and even depression. The frustration of not being able to recall once-familiar details or navigate commonplace tasks can erode self-esteem and diminish overall emotional well-being.

As cognitive function declines, there can be a shift in one's identity and sense of self. The person grappling with severe memory loss may find it challenging to recognize their own reflection, both figuratively and literally. This evolving self-awareness, coupled with potential mood swings and personality changes, can lead to a sense of disconnection from one's past and a reevaluation of one's present identity.

Is It Too Late? Embracing Hope in Memory Enhancement

While we are understanding severe memory loss, a common question lingers: Is it too late to reverse or improve the impacts of memory decline? It is a query often accompanied by a mix of concern and curiosity, especially for those who may have noticed the subtle signs of cognitive changes over time. The resounding answer is that it is never too late to embark on the journey of memory enhancement.

While it is true that for some individuals, certain aspects of memory loss may be inevitable due to factors such as aging or underlying health conditions, the capacity for memory improvement, reversal, or alleviation remains a viable and hopeful prospect. The human brain exhibits a remarkable degree of plasticity, allowing it to adapt and reorganize itself in response to new experiences and stimuli.

Engaging in activities specifically designed to stimulate cognitive function can yield positive results, even for individuals grappling with severe memory loss. These activities serve as mental exercises, fostering the growth and connections of neural pathways, ultimately contributing to enhanced cognitive abilities.

Moreover, the introduction of healthy lifestyle practices can play a pivotal role in mitigating memory decline. Proper nutrition, regular exercise, and sufficient sleep are all factors that influence brain health and contribute to overall well-being. Embracing these lifestyle adjustments can be a transformative step toward not only slowing the progression of memory loss but also improving cognitive function.

So, remember, while the journey of memory enhancement may require commitment and dedication, it is a journey well worth taking. By embracing the belief that it is never too late, individuals can foster a sense of agency and embark on a path of discovery, unlocking the potential for improved cognitive well-being and a more vibrant, fulfilling life.

Coping With Severe Memory Loss: Forgetting People

For individuals grappling with severe memory loss, the challenge of forgetting loved ones can be particularly poignant and emotionally taxing. It is an experience that echoes not only through the affected individual but also resonates with the family and friends witnessing the shifts in cognitive function. Understanding and navigating this facet of memory loss requires compassion, resilience, and the recognition that support and coping mechanisms can make a significant difference.

One effective strategy is the cultivation of a supportive environment. Loved ones and caregivers can play a crucial role in creating an atmosphere that encourages patience, understanding, and open communication. Establishing routines and maintaining consistency in interactions can provide a sense of stability for both the individual experiencing memory loss and those around them.

Moreover, fostering a rich sensory environment can serve as a valuable aid. Surrounding the individual with familiar scents, textures, and objects can trigger positive memories and create a comforting atmosphere. Photographs, memorabilia, and items with sentimental value can serve as anchors, offering a tangible connection to the past and the people within it.

In addition, embracing the power of music can be a remarkable coping mechanism. Music has a unique ability to evoke emotions and memories. Creating playlists featuring beloved tunes from the past can provide a powerful avenue for reminiscence, fostering moments of connection and joy.

It is essential to acknowledge that this chapter serves as a stepping stone toward practical solutions and engaging activities to aid in coping with severe memory loss, especially the challenge of forgetting loved ones.

Coping With Misplacing Things in the Maze of Memory Loss

Misplacing everyday items is a common frustration for many, but for those grappling with severe memory loss, it can be a persistent challenge that adds an extra layer of complexity to daily life. Losing keys, glasses, or even important documents can contribute to feelings of disorientation and anxiety. However, there are practical strategies that individuals can employ to cope with the vexing issue of misplacing things.

Establish Designated Spaces

Create specific, easily accessible places for frequently used items. Designate a spot for keys, a designated drawer for important documents, or a particular shelf for eyeglasses. Consistency in placing items in these designated spaces can help reduce the likelihood of misplacement.

Use Visual Reminders

Employ visual cues to trigger memory recall. For example, place colorful labels on drawers or containers to indicate their contents. Visual reminders act as prompts, aiding in the retrieval of information and reducing the chances of forgetting where an item is stored.

Create a Checklist

Develop a daily checklist for essential items and activities. This can serve as a mental guide and help maintain a routine. Regularly reviewing the checklist throughout the day provides visual reinforcement of tasks and reduces the likelihood of overlooking important details.

Utilize Technology

Leverage technology to assist in organization. Smartphone apps, smart home devices, and digital calendars can be valuable tools for setting reminders and keeping track of important events, appointments, and tasks.

Practice Mindfulness Techniques

Cultivate mindfulness to enhance present-moment awareness. Focusing on the current task or activity can reduce distractions and improve concentration, making it less likely to misplace items due to absentmindedness.

Engage in Memory-Boosting Activities

Participate in memory-enhancing activities and games. Chapter 6 will provide a variety of enjoyable exercises specifically designed to stimulate cognitive function and improve memory recall, offering practical solutions for coping with memory challenges.

Remember, the journey to cope with misplacing things is a process of exploration and adaptation. By incorporating these strategies into daily routines, you can create an environment that supports memory recall and fosters a sense of control, even in the face of severe memory loss.

Understanding the Widespread Impact of Severe Memory Loss

Beyond the realm of forgetting names or misplacing keys, severe memory loss can cast a profound shadow across various facets of a person's life. As we navigate this section on understanding memory decline, it is crucial to explore the broader spectrum of impacts, acknowledging the multifaceted challenges that individuals may encounter.

One significant area of impact is the disruption of daily activities. Severe memory loss can interfere with routine tasks such as cooking, shopping, or managing medications. The person may struggle to initiate or complete these activities, leading to a sense of frustration and a potential loss of independence. This impact reverberates through people's daily lives, shaping perceptions of self-efficacy and contributing to an evolving sense of identity.

Moreover, the social dimension of life is not immune to the effects of severe memory loss. Relationships with family and friends may transform as communication becomes more challenging. The person may withdraw from social interactions, feeling a sense of embarrassment or inadequacy. This shift can result in feelings of isolation and a diminishing quality of life.

Financial management is another area susceptible to the impacts of memory loss. Handling bills, budgeting, and making financial decisions may become formidable tasks. This can lead to stress, anxiety, and potential financial strain, accentuating the need for adaptive strategies to navigate this challenging terrain.

Coping Tools and Strategies

In the face of these challenges, it is essential to equip individuals with coping tools and strategies that empower them to navigate the impacts of severe memory loss. Below are some practical approaches to address these varied challenges.

Utilize Memory Aids

Integrate memory aids such as calendars, planners, and reminder apps into daily life. These tools can serve as external memory support, helping individuals stay organized and on top of their responsibilities.

Seek Professional Assistance

Engage the support of professionals, including healthcare providers, financial advisors, and social workers. These experts can offer tailored guidance and assistance in managing specific aspects impacted by memory loss.

Establish Support Networks

Foster a support network of family, friends, and caregivers. Open communication and shared responsibilities can alleviate the burden on the individual experiencing memory loss and create a collaborative approach to managing daily life.

Embrace Adaptive Techniques

Explore adaptive techniques for daily activities. This may include breaking tasks into smaller steps, using visual cues, or employing mnemonic devices to aid memory recall.

Participate in Cognitive Stimulation

Engage in regular cognitive stimulation activities and exercises. Chapter 6 will delve into a variety of enjoyable games and exercises proven to enhance cognitive function and memory recall.

The journey through memory loss is unique for each individual. Embrace a proactive and adaptable mindset, that will let you navigate these challenges with resilience and reclaim a sense of control and fulfillment in your life.

As we conclude this chapter on understanding severe memory loss, it is crucial to grasp that memory decline extends beyond mere forgetfulness, impacting daily activities, relationships, and overall well-being. By recognizing the signs, impacts, and diverse challenges associated with severe memory loss, we lay the foundation for the transformative journey ahead. This understanding is important in the broader context of our framework, as it sets the stage for the practical strategies and engaging activities we will explore in the next chapter, dedicated to managing severe memory loss. Join me as we go into a treasure trove of tools and exercises designed to empower and uplift, fostering cognitive resilience and a vibrant quality of life.

Chapter 6:

Managing Severe Memory Loss

Memory is an autumn leaf that murmurs a while in the wind and then is heard no more. –Kahlil Gibran

Now that we have laid the groundwork for understanding severe memory loss in earlier chapters, it is time to move on and learn to regain control, foster resilience, and discover joy despite the challenges that severe memory loss may bring. In the face of cognitive struggles, it is essential to recognize that there are activities, games, and strategies that not only mitigate the impact of memory loss but also actively contribute to enhancing cognitive function.

In this chapter, we will explore a diverse range of proven and enjoyable activities tailored specifically for those navigating severe memory loss. These activities are designed to engage the mind, spark memories, and promote a sense of accomplishment. Whether you are on a personal quest for cognitive improvement or assisting a loved one on this journey, these strategies offer a beacon of hope and empowerment.

Through the exploration of interactive games, stimulating exercises, and memory-enhancing techniques, we aim to show that there is always room for growth, connection, and joy, even in the face of significant memory challenges. By embracing these activities, we hope to not only counter the impact of memory loss but also create moments of fulfillment, laughter, and shared experiences.

Daily Planner Creation: A Roadmap to Unburdened Memory

Memory loss can sometimes feel like a dense fog, with the clarity of thoughts slipping away like elusive shadows. In the quest to manage severe memory loss, the creation and utilization of a daily planner can act as a guiding beacon, cutting through the haze and bringing a sense of order and purpose to each day.

The Power of a Daily Planner

A daily planner is more than just a notebook filled with appointments; it is a cognitive companion that assists in organizing thoughts, tasks, and goals. For seniors grappling with severe memory loss, a well-structured planner can be a source of reassurance and empowerment.

Refreshing Memory and Creating Mental Space

Think of a daily planner as an external memory bank. By jotting down tasks, appointments, and goals, you offload the burden from your internal memory, creating mental space for other important thoughts. It acts as a reliable reference point, ensuring that important details are not lost in the labyrinth of forgetfulness.

A daily planner is not only a tool for remembering but also a means to reclaim control over one's daily life. It provides a tangible structure to the seemingly chaotic landscape of memory challenges, offering a sense of stability and routine.

Crafting Your Personalized Daily Planner

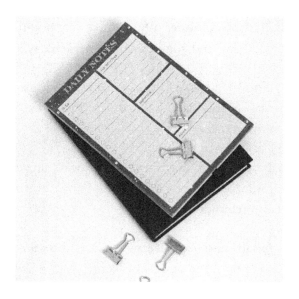

Creating a daily planner that suits your needs and preferences is a journey in itself. Here is a step-by-step guide to help you embark on this transformative process:

Step 1: Selecting the Right Planner

Choose a planner that resonates with you. Whether it is a traditional paper planner, a digital app, or a combination of both, the key is finding a format that aligns with your comfort level and lifestyle. Some may prefer the tactile experience of writing on paper, while others might appreciate the convenience of digital reminders.

Step 2: Define Your Planner Sections

Divide your planner into sections that cater to different aspects of your life. Common sections include:

- **Daily Schedule:** Outline your appointments, activities, and commitments for each day.

- **To-Do Lists:** Break down tasks into manageable steps. Prioritize them based on importance.

- **Notes and Reminders:** Allocate space for jotting down thoughts, important information, and reminders.

- **Goals and Achievements:** Dedicate a section to long-term and short-term goals. Celebrate small victories and progress.

Step 3: Establish a Daily Planning Routine

Consistency is key. Set aside a specific time each day to update and review your planner. This routine not only helps in reinforcing memories but also establishes a habit that contributes to overall cognitive well-being. Whether it is morning coffee and planning or an evening reflection, find a time that suits your daily rhythm.

Step 4: Use Visual Cues and Colors

Enhance the visual appeal of your planner by using colors and symbols. Differentiate between categories, highlight priorities, and create a visual roadmap that is easy to follow. Visual cues can serve as memory triggers, making it easier to recall information at a glance.

Step 5: Embrace Flexibility

Life is dynamic, and so should be your planner. Embrace flexibility by incorporating blank spaces for impromptu notes and adjustments. A rigid planner might add stress; instead, let it be a tool that adapts to your changing needs and circumstances.

Daily Planner Activity: Crafting Your Memory Oasis

Let us dive into a hands-on activity to kickstart your journey of daily planner creation. Find a comfortable and quiet space, gather your preferred materials, and let us begin.

Materials Needed

- **Planner of Your Choice:** Whether it is a physical notebook, a digital app, or a combination, ensure it suits your preferences.

- **Writing Tools:** Pens, markers, or stylus, depending on your chosen medium.

- **Sticky Notes or Tabs:** Optional, but useful for additional notes or marking important pages.

Activity Steps

Step 1: Reflect on Your Daily Routine

Take a moment to reflect on your typical day. What are your regular activities? When are your peak energy times? Identify the key elements that you want to incorporate into your daily planner.

Step 2: Choose Your Planner Sections

Based on your reflections, decide on the sections that will be most beneficial for you. If you have a lot of appointments, prioritize a detailed daily schedule. If you are working on specific goals, allocate space for tracking progress.

Step 3: Personalize With Colors and Symbols

Infuse your planner with personality by using colors and symbols. Assign specific colors to different categories or activities. For example, use green for health-related activities, blue for social engagements, and red for important deadlines.

Step 4: Set Up Your Daily Planning Routine

Establish a dedicated time for daily planning. It could be in the morning, before bedtime, or during a midday break. Consistency is key, so choose a time that aligns with your natural rhythms.

Step 5: Test and Adjust

Start using your planner and pay attention to how it influences your daily life. Does it help you remember important details? Are you feeling more in control? Do not hesitate to make adjustments as needed. Your planner is a dynamic tool that should evolve with you.

Reflection

Take a moment to reflect on the process. How did it feel to create a personalized daily planner? Did you discover any preferences or insights about your daily routine? Remember, this planner is not just a practical tool; it is a reflection of your unique journey and a testament to your resilience in managing memory challenges.

Memory Journaling: Nurturing the Past for a Flourishing Present

This creative endeavor not only serves as a means of preserving cherished moments but also becomes a therapeutic journey, fostering a profound connection with one's own history. Let us explore the significance of memory journaling and take a look at some prompts to guide you on a captivating voyage through their memories.

The Essence of Memory Journaling

Memory journaling is an intimate dance with the past, allowing individuals to capture fleeting moments, emotions, and experiences. As memory loss threatens to cloud the clarity of recollections, journaling becomes a sanctuary where memories can be revisited, cherished, and preserved.

Reading Through Memories

Imagine flipping through the pages of a carefully crafted memory journal—a kaleidoscope of moments etched in ink, each page holding a story, a feeling, a piece of the self. For seniors navigating severe memory loss, these journals become a bridge to the past, a tangible reminder of a life well-lived.

A Gift to Yourself and Others

Memory journaling is not only a gift to oneself but also to future generations. It serves as a legacy, offering insights into a personal history that may otherwise fade away. Sharing these written reflections with loved ones provides a unique opportunity for connection and understanding, fostering a sense of continuity and shared identity.

Getting Started With Memory Journaling

Embarking on a memory journaling journey requires nothing more than a notebook, a pen, and a willingness to explore the recesses of one's mind. Here is a guide to help you get started:

Step 1: Choose Your Journal

Select a journal that speaks to you—whether it is a leather-bound notebook, a digital journaling app, or a handmade creation. The key is to find something that resonates with your style and encourages you to return to its pages.

Step 2: Set the Mood

Create a conducive atmosphere for journaling. Find a comfortable and quiet space, perhaps with soft lighting and your favorite writing music. This helps create a sanctuary for reflection and introspection.

Step 3: Reflect on the Purpose

Before diving into the prompts, take a moment to reflect on why you want to engage in memory journaling. Is it to preserve moments for yourself? To share stories with loved ones? Establishing a clear purpose can guide your journaling journey.

Step 4: Embrace Openness

Approach memory journaling with an open heart and mind. It is not about perfection or chronological accuracy; it is about capturing the essence of the memory as you remember it. Embrace the beauty of imperfection.

Memory Journaling Prompts

Now, let us embark on a journey of self-discovery and reflection with these memory journaling prompts.

Feel free to explore each prompt at your own pace, allowing memories to flow naturally onto the pages of your journal.

- **The Earliest Memory:** Describe the first memory that comes to mind from your childhood.

- **Favorite Childhood Games:** Recount the games and activities you enjoyed as a child.

- **Family Traditions:** Share the traditions that held special significance in your family.

- **School Days:** Reflect on your favorite subjects, teachers, and memorable moments from your school days.

- **Celebrations and Holidays:** Write about memorable celebrations, holidays, and gatherings.

- **First Job Experience:** Recollect your first job experience, the challenges, and the lessons learned.

- **Romantic Moments:** Share special moments with your significant other or memorable romantic experiences.

- **Travel Adventures:** Write about your favorite travel destinations and the adventures you had.

- **Friendships:** Reflect on friendships that left a lasting impact on your life.

- **Achievements and Milestones:** Chronicle your proudest achievements and significant milestones.

- **Hobbies and Passions:** Explore your hobbies and passions, past and present.

- **Family Recipes:** Document cherished family recipes and the memories associated with them.

- **Unexpected Acts of Kindness:** Recall instances of unexpected kindness you have experienced or witnessed.

- **Pets and Animal Companions:** Share stories about pets or animals that have been a part of your life.

- **Learning Moments:** Write about experiences that taught you valuable life lessons.

- **Cultural Influences:** Explore the cultural influences that have shaped your identity.

- **Technology Transformations:** Reflect on how technology has evolved during your lifetime.

- **Memorable Quotes:** Share quotes or sayings that have inspired or resonated with you.

- **Weather Memories:** Recall significant weather events or moments tied to specific seasons.

- **Childhood Dreams:** Write about your aspirations and dreams as a child.

- **Changes in Your Hometown:** Document the transformations you have witnessed in your hometown.

- **Favorite Books and Films:** Explore the books and films that left a lasting impression on you.

- **Life Lessons From Elders:** Share wisdom passed down from older generations.

- **Adapting to Challenges:** Reflect on how you have navigated challenges and adapted over the years.

- **Favorite Childhood Foods:** Describe the flavors and aromas of your favorite childhood foods.

- **Unforgettable Smells:** Recall scents that evoke strong memories.

- **Musical Memories:** Document songs or musical genres that hold sentimental value.

- **Hidden Talents:** Share any hidden talents or skills you have discovered over the years.

- **Community Involvement:** Write about your involvement in community activities or causes.

- **Changes in Fashion:** Explore how fashion trends have changed during your lifetime.

- **Historical Events:** Reflect on your memories of significant historical events.

- **Technology Transformations:** Write about how advancements in technology have impacted your daily life.

- **Nature Escapes:** Describe moments spent in nature that left a lasting impression.

- **Mentors and Role Models:** Reflect on individuals who have inspired and influenced you.

- **Unexpected Adventures:** Recall spontaneous and unexpected adventures you have embarked on.

- **Treasured Keepsakes:** Write about keepsakes or mementos that hold sentimental value.

- **Life in Different Decades:** Explore how life has changed for you over different decades.

Remember that each prompt is a gateway to a treasure trove of experiences. Your memories are a unique mosaic that deserves to be celebrated and preserved. Use these prompts as sparks to ignite the flame of storytelling within you.

Through the act of memory journaling, you not only engage in a therapeutic exercise for your mind but also contribute to the preservation of your personal narrative. Your stories, reflections, and memories are the threads that weave the fabric of your life, creating a tapestry that deserves to be unfolded and admired.

Matching Games: Unveiling the Joy of Simplicity for Severe Memory Loss

Matching games, reminiscent of childhood play, emerge as delightful tools to engage the mind, improve memory in bits, and infuse moments of joy into the daily routine. Let us explore the benefits of matching games and take a look at a list of carefully selected games to enhance cognitive function with a gentle touch.

The Power of Matching Games

Matching games hold a special place in memory enhancement strategies, providing a playful and accessible way to stimulate cognitive processes. These games leverage the brain's pattern recognition abilities, offering a structured and enjoyable exercise for individuals dealing with severe memory challenges.

A Return to the Basics

As we navigate the complexities of memory loss, returning to the simplicity of matching games can be a nostalgic and effective approach. These games tap into fundamental cognitive functions, fostering a sense of accomplishment and satisfaction. The joy derived from successfully matching pairs not only boosts morale but also contributes to the overall well-being of people facing severe memory difficulties.

Fostering Concentration and Focus

Matching games require participants to concentrate and focus on visual cues, encouraging the brain to actively engage in the task at hand. This heightened attention can lead to improved concentration, a valuable skill in managing memory-related challenges.

Encouraging Social Interaction

Many matching games can be adapted for group play, providing an opportunity for social interaction. Engaging in these games with friends, family, or fellow seniors not only enhances the fun factor but also promotes a sense of connection and camaraderie.

Matching Games for Severe Memory Loss

Now, let us explore a list of matching games specifically designed for individuals facing very severe memory loss. These games are characterized by simplicity, visual clarity, and adaptability, making them accessible and enjoyable for everyone.

Picture Match

Match pairs of identical pictures.

Materials Needed

- A set of cards with simple, easily recognizable images (e.g., animals, objects). They should be large, easy-to-handle cards for better visibility.

How to Play

- Shuffle the cards and lay them face down.

- Participants take turns flipping two cards at a time, the purpose is to find matching pairs.

- When a pair is successfully matched, leave the cards face up. If not, flip them back face down.

- Continue until all pairs are matched.

Benefits

- Enhances visual recognition.

- Improves concentration and focus.

- Provides a gentle and enjoyable mental exercise.

Color Match

Match pairs of identical colors.

Materials Needed

- Color swatches or cards with different colored patterns

How to Play

- Place the color swatches/cards face down on the playing surface.

- Participants flip two cards at a time, aiming to find matching colors.

- If the colors match, leave the cards face up; if not, flip them back face down.

- Continue until all color pairs are matched.

Benefits

- Stimulates visual perception.

- Encourages color recognition.

- Fosters a sense of achievement.

Number Match

Match pairs of identical numbers.

Materials Needed

- Cards with large, clear numbers

How to Play

- Shuffle the cards and lay them face down.

- Participants turn over two cards at a time, aiming to find matching numbers.

- If the numbers match, leave the cards face up; unsuccessful attempts are flipped back face down.

- Continue until all number pairs are matched.

Benefits

- Enhances number recognition.

- Promotes cognitive engagement.

- Reinforces basic counting skills.

Word Match

Match pairs of identical words.

Materials Needed

- Cards with simple, easily readable words

How to Play

- Shuffle the cards and place them face down.

- Participants turn over two cards at a time, aiming to find matching words.

- Keep successful matches face up; flip unmatched cards back face down.

- Continue until all word pairs are matched.

Benefits
- Stimulates language recognition.

- Encourages reading and word association.

- Provides an enjoyable linguistic exercise.

Shape Match

Match pairs of identical shapes.

Materials Needed
- Cards with clear, simple shapes

How to Play
- Shuffle the cards and lay them face down.

- Participants flip two cards at a time, attempting to find matching shapes.

- Successful matches keep the cards face up, while unmatched cards are flipped back face down.

- Continue until all shape pairs are matched.

Benefits

- Enhances visual-spatial recognition.

- Encourages shape identification.

- Promotes a sense of accomplishment.

Memory Dominoes

Match pairs of identical dominoes.

Materials Needed

- Large domino pieces with clear, contrasting dots

How to Play

- Shuffle the domino pieces and arrange them face down.

- Participants turn over two dominoes at a time, aiming to find matching pairs.

- Successful matches keep the dominoes face up, while unmatched pieces are flipped back face down.

- Continue until all domino pairs are matched.

Benefits

- Enhances pattern recognition.

- Encourages strategic thinking.

- Offers a tactile and visually stimulating activity.

Texture Match

Match pairs of identical textures.

Materials Needed

- Cards or objects with distinct textures (e.g., smooth, rough, soft)

How to Play

- Arrange the texture cards or objects face down.

- Participants feel and explore two textures at a time, aiming to find matching pairs.

- Successful matches keep the cards or objects in view, while unmatched pairs are returned face down.

- Continue until all texture pairs are matched.

Benefits

- Stimulates tactile perception.

- Encourages sensory exploration.

- Provides a multisensory experience.

So you see, matching games, with their simplicity and adaptability, offer a delightful avenue for seniors facing severe memory loss to engage in cognitive exercises. These activities not only stimulate memory but also provide a platform for social interaction, fostering a sense of connection and joy.

As you explore these matching games, remember that the journey is as important as the destination. Embrace the moments of success, celebrate the joy of play, and savor the connections forged through these engaging activities.

Repetition Games: Harnessing the Power of Reinforcement for Memory Enhancement

When managing severe memory loss, repetition emerges as a potent ally. Repetition games, designed to reinforce information through repeated exposure, offer a structured and enjoyable way to enhance memory capacity.

The Science of Repetition

Repetition is a fundamental principle in memory enhancement. The process of repeating information helps strengthen neural pathways, making it easier for the brain to retrieve and retain that information. For seniors grappling with severe memory loss, incorporating repetition into cognitive activities becomes a valuable strategy to promote recall and reinforce key concepts.

Building Resilience Through Practice

Repetition is akin to practicing a skill—it builds resilience and familiarity. By engaging in repetition games, individuals not only enhance their memory but also develop a sense of confidence and mastery over the material. This approach fosters a positive feedback loop, encouraging continuous engagement with cognitive exercises.

Targeting Different Learning Styles

Repetition caters to various learning styles, accommodating both visual and auditory learners. Whether through visual cues, spoken words, or physical actions, repetition games provide a diverse range of stimuli that cater to individual preferences. This versatility is especially crucial in addressing the unique needs of seniors facing severe memory challenges.

Repetition Games for Severe Memory Loss

Now, let us delve into a curated list of repetition games designed to bolster memory retention and cognitive function for individuals with severe memory loss. These games are characterized by simplicity, adaptability, and the power to transform repetition into an enjoyable and engaging experience.

Word Chain

Create a chain of words by repeating and adding new words in sequence.

How to Play

- Start with a simple word (e.g., "sun").

- Each participant takes turns repeating the previous word and adding a new word to the chain (e.g., "sun," "flower," "butterfly").

- Continue the chain, with each participant recalling and adding to the sequence.

Benefits

- Enhances verbal memory.

- Encourages word association.

- Fosters group participation.

Pattern Recognition Cards

Recognize and remember patterns on a set of cards.

Materials Needed

- Cards with distinct patterns or images

How to Play

- Display a set of pattern cards.

- Participants observe the patterns for a set time.

- Cover the cards, and participants recall and replicate the patterns on blank cards.

- Increase difficulty by adding more cards or intricate patterns as the game progresses.

Benefits

- Stimulates visual memory.

- Encourages concentration and focus.

- Provides a tangible and visual memory exercise.

Musical Memory Challenge

Repeat and recall a sequence of musical notes or tones.

Materials Needed

- A simple musical instrument (e.g., xylophone, chimes).

- A chart indicating the musical notes.

How to Play

- Play a sequence of musical notes on the instrument.

- Participants listen and repeat the sequence using the same instrument.

- Increase the complexity of the sequence as participants become more comfortable.

- Encourage participants to take turns creating and repeating sequences.

Benefits

- Stimulates auditory memory.

- Enhances musical recognition.

- Offers a multisensory experience.

Number Recall Challenge

Repeat and recall a sequence of numbers.

How to Play

- Start with a simple sequence of numbers (e.g., 3-7-2).

- Participants repeat the sequence aloud.

- Gradually increase the length and complexity of the number sequences.

- Encourage participants to recall and repeat the sequences in reverse order.

Benefits

- Strengthens numerical memory.

- Enhances concentration and attention.

- Provides a structured numerical exercise.

Color Pattern Repetition

Replicate and extend a sequence of colors.

Materials Needed

- Colored cards or blocks

How to Play

- Display a sequence of colored cards or blocks.

- Participants replicate the sequence using the same colors.

- Gradually increase the length and complexity of the color sequences.

- Introduce variations, such as changing the order or adding new colors.

Benefits

- Enhances visual memory.

- Encourages color recognition.

- Provides a visually engaging exercise.

Daily Routine Reminder

Create and follow a daily routine with repeated activities.

How to Play

- Develop a simple daily routine chart with key activities (e.g., morning walk, reading time).

- Review the routine with participants, emphasizing the sequence of activities.

- Encourage participants to follow the routine daily, repeating the sequence of activities.

Benefits

- Establishes a structured daily routine.

- Reinforces memory through repetition.

- Promotes independence and organization.

Picture Sequence Storytelling

Recall and repeat the sequence of events in a picture story.

Materials Needed

- Picture cards that illustrate a simple story or sequence of events

How to Play

- Display the picture cards in a specific order to create a visual story.

- Participants observe the sequence and retell the story in their own words.

- Increase complexity by introducing additional picture cards or changing the story order.

- Encourage creative storytelling based on the visual cues.

Benefits

- Stimulates visual memory.

- Enhances narrative and storytelling skills.

- Fosters creativity and imagination.

Repetition games, with their structured and engaging nature, provide a valuable framework for memory enhancement among seniors facing severe memory challenges.

The activities outlined in this chapter not only reinforce neural pathways but also infuse the process of repetition with a sense of joy and accomplishment.

Strategies for Enhanced Memory Recall

Remembering people, places, and things becomes a crucial aspect of maintaining independence and a sense of connectedness. That is why I am going to introduce you to four activities designed to address specific challenges associated with recalling things, utilizing associative memory through mnemonics, and remembering common locations. These activities aim to empower seniors facing severe memory loss by providing practical and enjoyable tools to enhance memory recall.

Activity #1: Routine Planning

Planning Your Routine for Improved Memory Recall

Creating and following a routine can significantly improve the likelihood of remembering important tasks and activities. This activity involves planning and posting routines in prominent places to serve as visual reminders.

Steps

- Identify key activities.

- List the essential activities you engage in daily or weekly.

- Include tasks such as medication reminders, meal times, exercise routines, and social activities.

Create a Visual Routine

- Use a large piece of paper or a whiteboard to create a visual representation of your routine.

- Arrange the activities in a sequential order, highlighting specific times if necessary.

Color Code and Categorize

- Assign colors or symbols to different categories of activities (e.g., blue for health-related tasks, red for social activities).

- This visual coding enhances memory recall by associating colors with specific types of activities.

Place in Prominent Locations

- Post the visual routine in places where you spend a significant amount of time, such as the bedroom or kitchen.

- Ensure the routine is easily visible and accessible.

Review and Update

- Regularly review and update the routine as needed.

- Encourage family members or caregivers to be aware of the routine to provide additional support.

Benefits

- Provides a visual aid for daily planning.

- Enhances memory recall through routine reinforcement.

- Fosters independence and organization.

Activity #2: Facial Recognition

Practicing Facial Recognition With Movie or TV Characters

Facial recognition can be challenging, but engaging in activities that exercise this skill can lead to improvement. This activity involves using movie or TV characters as a fun and effective way to practice recognizing faces.

Steps

- Select movie or TV characters.

    ○ Choose a set of movie or TV characters with distinct features.

    ○ Aim for characters that participants may find interesting or entertaining.

- Create cards or flashcards.

    ○ Develop cards or flashcards featuring pictures of the selected characters.

    ○ Include the character's name on the back of each card.

- Practice regular sessions.

  - Conduct regular sessions where participants review the character cards.

  - Encourage them to memorize the names associated with each face.

- Organize quizzes and challenges.

  - Organize quizzes or challenges where participants identify characters from the cards.

  - Gradually increase the difficulty by introducing new characters or mixing up the cards.

- Discuss and share.

  - Facilitate discussions about the characters, their roles, and any memorable scenes.

  - This process helps reinforce memory through association.

Benefits
- Improves facial recognition skills.

- Utilizes entertainment to make the activity enjoyable.

- Encourages social interaction through shared discussions.

Activity #3: Associative Memory - Mnemonics

Creating Mnemonics for Memory Enhancement

Associative memory, particularly through the use of mnemonics, can significantly aid in remembering information. This activity challenges readers to create three mnemonic devices to practice and strengthen their associative memory.

Steps

- Understand mnemonics.

  ○ Explain the concept of mnemonics, which involves creating associations to aid memory.

  ○ Mnemonics can involve rhymes, acronyms, or vivid mental images.

- Identify three challenging items.

  - Choose three items or pieces of information that you often find challenging to remember. Examples could include names, numbers, or specific tasks.

- Create mnemonics.

  - Develop unique mnemonic devices for each chosen item.

  - For names, create a rhyme or association with a familiar word. For numbers, use an acronym or a memorable phrase.

- Practice regularly.

  - Incorporate these mnemonics into your daily routine.

  - Revisit and reinforce them regularly to strengthen the associations.

- Reflect on effectiveness.

  - Reflect on how well the mnemonics are working for you.

o Adjust or create new mnemonics if needed.

Benefits

● Enhances associative memory through creative associations.

● Provides a personalized and adaptable memory strategy.

● Encourages active engagement with memory enhancement techniques.

Activity #4: Remembering Location

Remembering common locations is vital for independence and navigation. This interactive game involves engaging the senses, basic mnemonics, and more to enhance memory recall of frequently visited places.

Steps

● Select common locations.

o Identify three to five common locations you visit regularly (e.g., a grocery store, a friend's house, or a local park).

- Create a memory map.

  - Mentally map out the key features of each location.

  - Note distinct landmarks, colors, or smells associated with each place.

- Engage the senses.

  - Visit each location or use images to engage the senses.

  - Pay attention to the sounds, smells, and visual cues in each environment.

- Create mnemonic associations.

  - Develop simple mnemonic associations for each location. For example, associate the grocery store with a bright red sign or a favorite scent.

- Narrate the journey.

  - Practice narrating the journey from one location to another.

  - Use the mnemonics and sensory associations to reinforce memory.

- Interactive driving or map game.

  - If there is an opportunity, engage in an interactive driving or map game.

  - Challenge yourself to recall and navigate to the selected locations.

Benefits

- Enhances spatial memory and navigation skills.

- Encourages sensory engagement for a multi-sensory memory experience.

- Utilizes mnemonics to reinforce memory associations.

These activities aim to provide practical and enjoyable tools for seniors facing severe memory challenges. Incorporating these activities into daily routines can contribute to a holistic approach to managing severe memory loss.

In this chapter on managing severe memory loss, we explored activities such as routine planning, facial recognition, associative memory through mnemonics, and games for remembering locations. These strategies, rooted in simplicity and engagement, aim to empower seniors facing memory challenges with practical tools and joyful experiences. As an integral part of our broader framework for enhancing cognitive function, this chapter emphasizes the significance of addressing specific aspects of memory recall to create a holistic approach toward improvement.

Understanding that memory enhancement is a multifaceted journey, our next chapter moves into the essential roles of diet, nutrition, and exercise in promoting cognitive well-being. We will explore how adopting a healthy lifestyle can contribute to the overall goal of preserving and enhancing memory function. Get ready to nourish both body and mind as we embark on the next phase of our exploration into the realms of well-balanced living and cognitive vitality.

Chapter 7:

Diet, Nutrition, and Exercise

Our memory is like a shop in the window of which there is now one, now another photograph of the same person. And as a rule the most recent exhibit remains for some time the only one to be seen. –Marcel Proust

By now, you have discovered a treasure trove of engaging games, activities, and coping skills that promise to be your companions on this exciting cognitive fitness adventure. Armed with these tools, you are now ready to explore simple lifestyle solutions that can have a profound impact on memory improvement.

Here, we will explore the powerful realms of diet, nutrition, and exercise—three pillars that not only contribute to overall well-being but play a crucial role in sharpening and preserving our mental faculties. As we navigate through these lifestyle enhancements, you will find practical, enjoyable, and proven strategies tailored to meet the unique needs of seniors who are keen on boosting their memory and cognitive abilities.

The approach is rooted in the understanding that a holistic lifestyle, encompassing mind and body, is key to unlocking the full potential of your cognitive functions. So, let us embark on this exciting journey together, starting with the foundations of a well-nourished body and an active, rejuvenated mind. Get ready to embrace the benefits that a thoughtful diet and exercise regimen can bring to your life, enhancing not only your memory but your overall quality of life. The path to cognitive vitality begins with the choices we make every day, and I am here to guide you every step of the way.

Nourishing Your Mind: The Impact of Nutrition on Memory

One of the most crucial elements we encounter in this topic is the role of nutrition in preserving and improving memory. The adage "You are what you eat" takes on a profound significance when it comes to the workings of our brain.

Now, let us explore the symbiotic relationship between nutrition and memory, unraveling how a well-balanced diet can become a powerful ally in the pursuit of cognitive vitality.

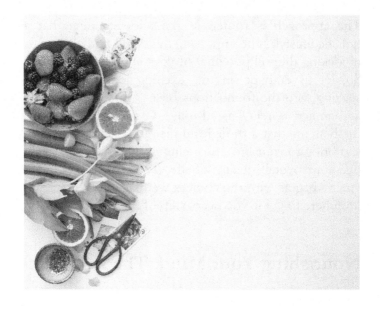

The Brain's Culinary Palette

Our brains require a diverse range of nutrients to function optimally. Imagine your brain as a gourmet chef crafting intricate dishes—each nutrient playing a unique role in supporting cognitive functions, with memory at the forefront of the menu.

Omega-3 Fatty Acids: The Brain's Best Friend

Omega-3 fatty acids found abundantly in fatty fish like salmon, flaxseeds, and walnuts, are instrumental in building and maintaining the structure of brain cells. These essential fatty acids contribute to the development of cell membranes, ensuring smooth communication between brain cells, which is fundamental for memory consolidation.

Antioxidants: Guardians Against Oxidative Stress

Berries, dark chocolate, and green leafy vegetables are rich sources of antioxidants, which act as guardians against oxidative stress. The brain, highly susceptible to oxidative damage, benefits from these antioxidants that neutralize harmful free radicals, preserving cognitive functions, including memory.

Vitamins and Minerals: Micronutrients for Cognitive Health

Essential vitamins such as B-complex vitamins (B6, B12, and folic acid) and minerals like zinc and magnesium play pivotal roles in cognitive health. B vitamins are crucial for the production of neurotransmitters, the brain's chemical messengers, while minerals support overall brain function. Incorporating a variety of fruits, vegetables, whole grains, and lean proteins ensures a rich supply of these micronutrients.

The Gut-Brain Connection

Beyond individual nutrients, we delve into the fascinating realm of the gut-brain connection. Emerging research suggests that the health of our gut microbiota, the trillions of microorganisms residing in our digestive tract, profoundly influences cognitive function, including memory.

Probiotics: Cultivating a Healthy Microbial Ecosystem

Foods rich in probiotics, such as yogurt, kefir, and fermented vegetables, foster a thriving community of beneficial bacteria in the gut. This microbial ecosystem, often referred to as the "second brain," communicates with the central nervous system, influencing cognitive processes. A balanced gut microbiome has been linked to improved memory and reduced cognitive decline.

Prebiotics: Nourishing the Microbial Garden

Prebiotics, found in foods like garlic, onions, and bananas, serve as the nourishment for beneficial gut bacteria. By including prebiotics in your diet, you cultivate a fertile ground for these microorganisms to flourish, indirectly supporting cognitive health and memory.

Crafting Your Memory-Boosting Plate

Now that we have explored the building blocks of a memory-friendly diet, let us discuss practical steps to incorporate these elements into your meals.

- **Mindful Eating—Savoring the Experience:** Slow down, engage your senses, and savor each bite. Mindful eating not only enhances your appreciation for food but also allows your brain to register the experience, promoting better memory recall.

- **Colorful Variety—A Spectrum of Nutrients:** Embrace a rainbow on your plate. Each color in fruits and vegetables represents a unique set of nutrients. A diverse, colorful diet ensures you receive a broad spectrum of vitamins, minerals, and antioxidants, providing comprehensive support for your cognitive functions.

- **Hydration—Nourishing Your Brain With Water:** Staying adequately hydrated is fundamental for optimal brain function. Dehydration can impair concentration and memory. Make water your beverage of choice and consider incorporating hydrating foods like watermelon and cucumber into your meals.

Personalizing Your Nutritional Journey

Consider consulting with a healthcare professional or a registered dietitian to tailor your diet to your specific requirements. Factors such as age, existing health conditions, and personal preferences play a crucial role in determining the most suitable nutritional approach for you.

In the quest for cognitive enhancement, remember that small, sustainable changes to your diet can yield significant benefits over time. As you embark on this nutritional journey, relish the opportunity to nourish not only your body but also your mind. The culinary choices you make today could be the key to unlocking a future filled with vibrant memories and cognitive vitality.

Energizing Your Mind: The Transformative Power of Exercise on Memory

The relationship between physical activity and cognitive health, particularly memory improvement, is a topic that continues to captivate researchers and health enthusiasts alike.

The Exercise-Memory Connection

Brain-Derived Neurotrophic Factor (BDNF)

At the heart of the exercise-memory connection lies a fascinating protein called brain-derived neurotrophic factor (BDNF). Exercise triggers the release of BDNF, often referred to as the "miracle growth for the brain." This protein plays a crucial role in promoting the growth, survival, and differentiation of neurons, particularly in regions of the brain associated with learning and memory.

Improved Blood Flow

Engaging in regular physical activity enhances blood flow throughout the body, including the brain. Improved circulation ensures a steady supply of oxygen and nutrients to brain cells, fostering an environment conducive to optimal cognitive function. This increased blood flow is particularly beneficial for memory-related regions of the brain, such as the hippocampus.

Neurogenesis

Contrary to the long-held belief that the adult brain does not generate new cells, recent research suggests that exercise promotes neurogenesis, the growth of new neurons. The hippocampus, a key player in memory formation, experiences a boost in cell production through regular physical activity, providing a structural foundation for improved memory.

Choosing the Right Exercise for Memory Enhancement

Not all exercises are created equal when it comes to memory improvement.

While any form of physical activity is beneficial, certain types of exercises offer specific advantages for cognitive health.

- **Aerobic Exercise—Boosting Brain Power:** Aerobic exercises, such as brisk walking, jogging, swimming, and dancing, have been consistently linked to improved memory and cognitive function. These activities elevate heart rate and increase oxygen intake, creating an optimal environment for BDNF release and neurogenesis.

- **Strength Training—Building a Resilient Brain:** Resistance or strength training exercises, involving activities like weightlifting or resistance band workouts, contribute to overall brain health. Building and maintaining muscle mass is associated with better cognitive performance, including memory retention.

- **Mind-Body Exercises—The Harmony of Body and Mind:** Mind-body exercises, such as yoga and tai chi, offer a unique blend of physical activity and mental focus. These practices have been shown to enhance memory and cognitive abilities by promoting relaxation, reducing stress, and improving overall brain function.

Exercise as a Memory Booster in Everyday Life

Incorporating exercise into your daily routine does not necessarily mean embarking on a rigorous fitness regimen. The efforts can yield significant benefits.

Daily Walks: A Step Toward Memory Enhancement

Take a daily stroll in nature or around your neighborhood. Walking not only promotes physical health but also provides a mental break, allowing your brain to recharge and consolidate memories.

Stair Climbing: Elevate Your Memory

Opt for stairs instead of elevators whenever possible. Climbing stairs engages multiple muscle groups and gets your heart pumping, contributing to improved blood flow and memory function.

Dance: Rhythmic Memories

Dance to your favorite tunes. Whether it is a solo dance party in your living room or joining a dance class, the rhythmic movements and coordination involved in dancing stimulate various regions of the brain linked to memory.

Building Sustainable Exercise Habits

As we age, it becomes increasingly vital to cultivate exercise habits that are not only effective but also sustainable. Here are some tips for integrating exercise into your routine:

- **Find Activities You Enjoy—Making Exercise Fun:** Choose activities that bring you joy. Whether it is gardening, swimming, or playing a sport, enjoyment is key to maintaining a consistent exercise routine.

- **Socialize Through Exercise—Combining Pleasure and Connection:** Engage in group exercises or classes. Socializing while exercising adds an extra layer of motivation and enjoyment, making it more likely that you will stick to your routine.

- **Gradual Progression—Start Small, Aim Big:** Begin with manageable activities and gradually increase intensity. Consistency is more important than intensity, and establishing a routine that you can maintain over time is key to reaping the cognitive benefits of exercise.

Consultation and Safety Considerations

Before starting a new exercise regimen, especially for individuals with existing health conditions, it is advisable to consult with a healthcare professional. They can provide personalized guidance and ensure that the chosen activities align with your health status and goals.

A Holistic Approach to Memory Enhancement

In the world of cognitive vitality, exercise emerges as a formidable ally, offering not only physical well-being but also a sharpened, resilient memory. As you embark on your journey toward a more active lifestyle, relish the notion that every step, every stretch, and every movement is a gift to your brain. The memories you create during your exercise endeavors may just be as enduring as the cognitive benefits they bring. So, lace up your sneakers, embrace the joy of movement, and witness the transformative power of exercise on your memory and overall well-being.

Culinary Alchemy: Nutrients for Memory Enhancement

Just as a well-composed song requires a great blend of instruments, our brain needs diverse and synergistic contributions of various nutrients.

DHA (Docosahexaenoic Acid): Building Blocks of Memory

DHA, a type of omega-3 fatty acid, is a crucial component of cell membranes in the brain. It contributes to the fluidity and flexibility of cell membranes, supporting efficient communication between neurons. Including fatty fish like salmon, mackerel, and trout in your diet provides a direct source of DHA, promoting memory improvement and cognitive resilience.

EPA (Eicosapentaenoic Acid): Reducing Inflammation

EPA, another omega-3 fatty acid, exerts anti-inflammatory effects on the brain. Chronic inflammation has been linked to cognitive decline, and EPA's anti-inflammatory properties contribute to a brain environment conducive to memory retention.

Incorporate fish oil supplements or algae-based omega-3 supplements if fish consumption is limited.

Vitamin C: Citrus Elixirs for Cognitive Vitality

Citrus fruits, strawberries, and bell peppers are excellent sources of vitamin C. This antioxidant scavenges free radicals, protecting brain cells from oxidative damage. A diet rich in vitamin C supports overall cognitive health and memory retention.

Vitamin E: Nuts, Seeds, and Leafy Greens

Nuts, seeds, and leafy green vegetables are packed with vitamin E, a potent antioxidant that safeguards cell membranes in the brain. Including almonds, sunflower seeds, and spinach in your diet contributes to the defense against oxidative stress, promoting memory improvement.

B6 (Pyridoxine): Unlocking Neurotransmitter Potential

Bananas, avocados, and poultry are rich sources of vitamin B6. This vitamin is involved in the production of neurotransmitters such as serotonin and dopamine, which play key roles in mood regulation and memory enhancement.

B12 (Cobalamin): Protecting Cognitive Resilience

Vitamin B12 is vital for the maintenance of nerve cells and the formation of myelin, the protective sheath around nerves. Found in animal products like meat, fish, and dairy, B12 contributes to cognitive resilience and memory improvement, particularly in seniors.

B9 (Folic Acid): Guarding Against Cognitive Decline

Leafy green vegetables, legumes, and fortified cereals provide ample folic acid. This B vitamin is crucial for DNA synthesis and repair and has been associated with a reduced risk of cognitive decline. Including folic acid in your diet supports overall brain health and memory function.

Zinc: Memory's Gatekeeper

Zinc is involved in the regulation of synaptic function, supporting communication between neurons. Oysters, beef, and pumpkin seeds are rich sources of zinc. Including these foods in your diet contributes to the gatekeeping role of zinc in memory enhancement.

Magnesium: Nurturing Neuronal Connections

Magnesium participates in synaptic plasticity, the ability of neurons to adapt and strengthen connections. Leafy green vegetables, nuts, and whole grains are excellent sources of magnesium. Including magnesium-rich foods supports the nurturing of neuronal connections, contributing to improved memory.

Mediterranean Diet: A Symphony of Cognitive Support

The Mediterranean diet, rich in fruits, vegetables, whole grains, fish, and healthy fats, has been consistently associated with cognitive benefits. This dietary pattern provides a holistic approach to memory improvement, emphasizing a balance of nutrients and antioxidants.

Hydration: Water for Cognitive Quenching

Staying well-hydrated is fundamental for optimal cognitive function. Dehydration can impair concentration and memory. Make water your beverage of choice and consider incorporating hydrating foods like watermelon and cucumber into your meals.

Personalizing Your Memory-Boosting Plate

As you embark on the journey of memory enhancement through nutrition, keep in mind that personalization is key. Factors such as individual health conditions, dietary preferences, and cultural considerations influence the most suitable approach for your unique needs.

Consultation With Healthcare Professionals: Tailoring Nutritional Strategies

Before making significant changes to your diet, especially if you have existing health conditions, consider consulting with healthcare professionals or registered dietitians. They can provide personalized guidance based on your health status and help you tailor your nutritional strategy for optimal memory improvement.

Gradual Changes for Sustainable Impact

Implementing small, gradual changes to your diet is more sustainable than attempting radical transformations. Aim for variety, balance, and moderation in your food choices, fostering a long-term commitment to memory-friendly nutrition.

Cultivating Eating Habits for Nutrient Absorption and Improved Memory

Cultivating mindful eating habits not only supports optimal nutrient absorption but also contributes to improved memory retention. Let us explore 15 habits that readers can adopt while eating, creating a synergistic environment for a nourished body and a sharpened mind.

Mindful Awareness Before Meals: A Prelude to Nourishment

Begin your meals with a moment of mindful awareness. Take a few deep breaths, appreciate the colors and aromas of your food, and express gratitude for the nourishment about to be received. This brief pause sets the stage for a more intentional and mindful eating experience.

Balanced Plate: A Symphony of Nutrients

Strive for a balanced plate that includes a variety of colors, textures, and nutrients. Aim to incorporate fruits, vegetables, lean proteins, whole grains, and healthy fats into your meals. This diverse array of foods ensures a comprehensive nutrient profile, supporting both overall health and memory improvement.

Chew Thoroughly: The Art of Mindful Mastication

Slow down and savor each bite. Chewing thoroughly not only aids in digestion but also allows your brain to register the flavors and textures of your food. This mindful mastication promotes a sense of satisfaction, reducing the likelihood of overeating.

Hydrate Wisely: Water as a Companion

Stay hydrated by sipping water throughout your meals. Adequate hydration supports digestion and nutrient absorption. Opt for water over sugary beverages, as excessive sugar intake has been linked to cognitive decline.

Optimal Meal Timing: Syncing With Circadian Rhythms

Align your meals with your body's natural circadian rhythms. Aim for regular meal times to promote a stable energy supply to the brain. Consistent meal timing can contribute to improved cognitive function and memory retention.

Include Healthy Fats: Brain's Fuel Source

Incorporate sources of healthy fats, such as avocados, nuts, seeds, and olive oil, into your meals. These fats provide essential fatty acids that support brain structure and function. Including healthy fats in your diet contributes to improved memory and cognitive health.

Limit Processed Foods: Minimizing Cognitive Distractions

Minimize the intake of processed and highly refined foods. These often contain additives and preservatives that may have negative effects on cognitive function. Opt for whole, unprocessed foods to provide your brain with the nutrients it needs for optimal performance.

Embrace Probiotics: Gut-Brain Symbiosis

Include probiotic-rich foods, such as yogurt, kefir, and fermented vegetables, to foster a healthy gut microbiome. The gut-brain connection is significant in cognitive health, and a balanced gut contributes to improved memory and overall well-being.

Plan Balanced Snacks: Sustaining Cognitive Energy

Plan nutrient-rich snacks between meals to sustain cognitive energy levels. Opt for snacks that combine protein, fiber, and healthy fats to provide a steady release of energy. Nuts, fruits, and yogurt with berries are excellent options for memory-friendly snacks.

Moderate Portion Sizes: Mindful Moderation

Practice portion control to avoid overeating. Use smaller plates, listen to your body's hunger and fullness cues, and be mindful of portion sizes. Consuming moderate amounts allows for better digestion and nutrient absorption.

Eat in a Calm Environment: Tranquil Digestion

Create a calm and peaceful environment for meals. Minimize distractions, such as television or excessive noise, to allow your focus to be on the sensory experience of eating. A tranquil environment promotes optimal digestion and nutrient absorption.

Include Memory-Boosting Herbs: Culinary Cognitive Support

Integrate memory-boosting herbs into your meals. Herbs like rosemary, thyme, and sage have been associated with cognitive benefits. These flavorful additions not only enhance the taste of your dishes but also contribute to improved memory retention.

Diverse Protein Sources: Building Cognitive Blocks

Diversify your protein sources to include fish, poultry, lean meats, beans, and legumes. Proteins provide the building blocks for neurotransmitters, supporting optimal brain function and memory enhancement.

Limit Added Sugars: Sweetness in Moderation

Be mindful of added sugars in your diet. Excessive sugar intake has been linked to cognitive decline and may impair memory function. You can use natural sweeteners like honey.

Reflect on Satisfaction: Gratitude for Nourishment

Conclude your meals with a moment of reflection. Acknowledge the nourishment you have received, and cultivate a sense of gratitude for the flavors and nutrients that contribute to your well-being. This mindful reflection enhances the overall eating experience.

As you incorporate these mindful eating habits into your daily routine, remember that the journey toward memory enhancement is a gradual and personalized process.

By adopting these habits, you not only create an environment conducive to nutrient absorption but also lay the foundation for improved memory retention. Mindful dining is not just about what you eat but how you eat, and these habits offer a holistic approach to nourishing both your body and your mind.

Delicious Brain Foods for Enhanced Memory

This section is dedicated to exploring dishes that incorporate stellar brain foods—ingredients rich in nutrients proven to enhance cognitive function and memory retention. Let us begin a flavorful adventure that not only tantalizes the taste buds but also fuels the mind.

Salmon Avocado Salad

Ingredients

- Fresh salmon fillets

- Avocado

- Leafy greens (spinach, arugula)

- Cherry tomatoes

- Olive oil and lemon dressing

Why It Is Stellar for Memory

- Salmon provides omega-3 fatty acids, particularly DHA, which support brain structure and function.

- Avocado contributes healthy fats and antioxidants, promoting optimal blood flow to the brain.

- Leafy greens supply essential vitamins and minerals for overall cognitive health.

Blueberry Walnut Oatmeal: Antioxidant-Rich Breakfast

Ingredients

- Oats

- Blueberries

- Chopped walnuts

- Cinnamon

- Greek yogurt (optional)

Why It Is Stellar for Memory

- Blueberries are rich in antioxidants, specifically anthocyanins, which have been linked to improved memory.

- Walnuts provide omega-3 fatty acids and antioxidants, supporting brain health.

- Oats offer complex carbohydrates for sustained energy, crucial for cognitive function.

Quinoa Spinach Stuffed Peppers: Nutrient-Packed Delight

Ingredients

- Quinoa

- Spinach

- Bell peppers

- Feta cheese

- Cherry tomatoes

Why It Is Stellar for Memory

- Quinoa is a whole grain rich in B vitamins, essential for neurotransmitter function.

- Spinach provides iron and folate, supporting cognitive function and reducing the risk of cognitive decline.

- Feta cheese adds a dose of calcium, crucial for neuronal health.

Grilled Chicken and Broccoli Stir-Fry: Protein-Packed Brain Fuel

Ingredients

- Chicken breast

- Broccoli florets

- Bell peppers

- Garlic and ginger

- Soy sauce

Why It Is Stellar for Memory

- Chicken is a lean protein source, supplying amino acids necessary for neurotransmitter synthesis.

- Broccoli contains vitamin K and choline, supporting brain health and memory.

- Soy sauce adds a savory touch and provides antioxidants.

Sweet Potato and Kale Frittata: Vitamin-Rich Brunch

Ingredients

- Sweet potatoes

- Kale

- Eggs

- Onion and garlic

- Feta cheese (optional)

Why It Is Stellar for Memory

- Sweet potatoes offer beta-carotene, converted into vitamin A, crucial for cognitive function.

- Kale is rich in vitamins K and C, supporting brain health.

- Eggs provide choline, essential for neurotransmitter production.

Chia Seed Pudding With Berries: Omega-3 Dessert

Ingredients

- Chia seeds

- Almond milk

- Mixed berries

- Honey or maple syrup

Why It Is Stellar for Memory

- Chia seeds are packed with fiber and antioxidants.

- Berries provide anthocyanins and vitamin C, contributing to improved cognitive function.

- Almond milk adds a creamy texture and supplies vitamin E.

Mediterranean Lentil Salad: Mediterranean Memory Boost

Ingredients

- Lentils

- Cherry tomatoes

- Cucumber

- Red onion

- Feta cheese

- Olive oil and lemon dressing

Why It Is Stellar for Memory
- Lentils are rich in folate and iron, supporting cognitive health.

- Tomatoes provide lycopene, an antioxidant associated with cognitive benefits.

- Olive oil adds monounsaturated fats, beneficial for brain health.

Turkey and Avocado Wrap: Nutrient-Packed Lunch

Ingredients
- Turkey slices

- Avocado

- Whole-grain wrap

- Spinach leaves

- Tomato slices

Why It Is Stellar for Memory
- Turkey is a lean protein source, supplying amino acids for neurotransmitter synthesis.

- Avocados contribute healthy fats and vitamin K for brain health.

- Whole-grain wrap provides complex carbohydrates for sustained energy.

Cauliflower and Broccoli Gratin: Cruciferous Comfort Food

Ingredients
- Cauliflower and broccoli florets

- Gruyere or cheddar cheese

- Milk or cream

- Garlic and nutmeg

Why It Is Stellar for Memory

- Cauliflower and broccoli belong to the cruciferous family, associated with cognitive benefits.

- Cheese provides vitamin B12 and calcium, crucial for brain health.

- Nutmeg adds a warm flavor and has cognitive-enhancing properties.

Pumpkin Seed Trail Mix: Nutrient-Packed Snack

Ingredients

- Pumpkin seeds

- Almonds

- Dried cranberries

- Dark chocolate chips

Why It Is Stellar for Memory

- Pumpkin seeds are rich in magnesium and zinc, supporting cognitive function.

- Almonds provide vitamin E, an antioxidant associated with memory improvement.

- Dark chocolate contains flavonoids, linked to enhanced cognitive performance.

Lemon Garlic Baked Salmon: Citrusy Omega-3 Delight

Ingredients
- Salmon fillets

- Lemon

- Garlic

- Fresh herbs (dill, parsley)

- Olive oil

Why It Is Stellar for Memory
- Salmon offers omega-3 fatty acids, promoting optimal brain function and memory improvement.

- Lemon provides vitamin C, enhancing the absorption of iron from the salmon.

- Garlic adds flavor and contains antioxidants with potential cognitive benefits.

Brussels Sprouts and Bacon Hash: Cruciferous Comfort Food

Ingredients
- Brussels sprouts

- Bacon

- Onion

- Garlic

- Parmesan cheese (optional)

Why It Is Stellar for Memory
- Brussels sprouts are rich in vitamins K and C, supporting cognitive health.

- Bacon provides choline and B vitamins essential for neurotransmitter synthesis.

- Parmesan cheese adds a savory touch and contributes to calcium intake.

Berry and Almond Smoothie Bowl: Antioxidant-Packed Breakfast

Ingredients

- Mixed berries (strawberries, blueberries, raspberries)

- Almond milk

- Greek yogurt

- Almond butter

- Granola and chia seeds for topping

Why It Is Stellar for Memory

- Berries supply antioxidants, including anthocyanins, linked to improved cognitive function.

- Almond butter offers healthy fats and vitamin E, supporting brain health.

- Greek yogurt provides protein and probiotics for gut-brain health.

Tomato Basil Quinoa Salad: Mediterranean Memory Marvel

Ingredients

- Quinoa

- Cherry tomatoes

- Fresh basil

- Feta cheese

- Balsamic vinaigrette

Why It Is Stellar for Memory

- Quinoa is rich in B vitamins, essential for neurotransmitter function.

- Tomatoes provide lycopene, an antioxidant associated with cognitive benefits.

- Basil adds a burst of flavor and has anti-inflammatory properties.

Cinnamon Apple Baked Oatmeal: Spiced Memory Magic

Ingredients

- Rolled oats

- Apples

- Cinnamon

- Almond milk

- Maple syrup

Why It Is Stellar for Memory

- Oats provide complex carbohydrates for sustained energy and cognitive support.

- Apples offer fiber and antioxidants, contributing to overall brain health.

- Cinnamon adds a warm flavor and has cognitive benefits.

As you explore these delicious dishes, remember that the key to optimizing memory through nutrition lies not in individual ingredients alone but in the harmonious combination of nutrient-rich foods. Embrace the joy of culinary experimentation, savor the flavors of wholesome ingredients, and relish the knowledge that each bite contributes to the nourishment of both body and mind.

Incorporating these brain-boosting foods into your regular meals not only supports memory improvement but also transforms the act of eating into a delightful and purposeful experience. Whether it is a salmon avocado salad, a blueberry walnut oatmeal, or a pumpkin seed trail mix, every dish can be a flavorful step toward cognitive vitality.

Unlocking Cognitive Benefits Through Exercise

The symbiotic relationship between regular physical activity and optimal brain health has been well-established through scientific research. Let us explore 10 physical activities that not only invigorate the body but also stimulate the mind, fostering a harmonious balance that promotes cognitive vitality.

Brisk Walking: The Gateway to Cognitive Fitness

How to do it

- Find a comfortable walking pace.

- Swing your arms naturally as you walk.

- Maintain an upright posture.

Why It Is Beneficial for Memory
- Brisk walking increases heart rate, promoting better blood flow to the brain.

- It stimulates the release of neurotransmitters that enhance mood and cognitive function.

- Regular walking has been associated with improved memory and cognitive performance.

Jogging or Running: Cardiovascular Boost for the Brain

How to do it
- Start with a gentle jog and gradually increase intensity.

- Use proper running shoes for support.

- Pay attention to your form to minimize the impact on joints.

Why It Is Beneficial for Memory

- Jogging or running elevates heart rate, improving blood flow to the brain.

- It stimulates the release of brain-derived neurotrophic factor (BDNF), promoting neuroplasticity and memory improvement.

- Cardiovascular exercise has been linked to a reduced risk of cognitive decline.

Yoga: Mind-Body Harmony for Memory Enhancement

How to do it

- Engage in yoga poses that promote balance.

- Incorporate mindful breathing and meditation techniques.

- Attend a yoga class or follow tutorials online.

Why It Is Beneficial for Memory

- Yoga combines physical movement with mindfulness, reducing stress and enhancing overall brain function.

- Certain yoga poses stimulate blood flow to the brain, promoting cognitive health.

- Mind-body practices have been associated with improved memory and attention.

Dance: Rhythmic Memory Boost

How to do it

- Choose a dance style you enjoy, such as salsa, ballroom, or hip-hop.

- Dance to your favorite music at home or join a dance class.

- Focus on rhythmic movements and coordination.

Why It Is Beneficial for Memory

- Dance engages multiple cognitive processes, including memory, attention, and spatial awareness.

- Rhythmic movements can enhance coordination and motor skills, supporting brain health.

- Social dance activities provide an additional layer of cognitive stimulation.

Strength Training: Building a Resilient Mind and Body

How to do it

- Use resistance bands, weights, or bodyweight exercises.

- Include compound exercises targeting major muscle groups.

- Gradually increase intensity and resistance over time.

Why It Is Beneficial for Memory

- Strength training promotes the release of growth factors that support brain health.

- Building and maintaining muscle mass is associated with better cognitive function.

- Resistance exercises contribute to overall physical well-being, creating a foundation for cognitive vitality.

Tai Chi: Flowing Movements for Cognitive Harmony

How to do it

- Learn and practice the slow, flowing movements of tai chi.

- Focus on deep and controlled breathing.

- Attend tai chi classes or follow instructional videos.

Why It Is Beneficial for Memory

- Tai chi combines physical exercise with mindfulness, reducing stress and promoting relaxation.

- The rhythmic movements enhance coordination and balance, supporting brain health.

- Regular practice has been associated with improved cognitive function and memory.

Pilates: Core Strength for Cognitive Stability

How to do it

- Engage in Pilates exercises that target core muscles.

- Use a mat or Pilates equipment for added resistance.

- Focus on controlled movements and proper breathing.

Why It Is Beneficial for Memory

- Pilates emphasizes core strength, which is integral for overall stability and balance.

- Controlled movements enhance body awareness and coordination, supporting cognitive function.

- Regular Pilates practice contributes to improved posture, reducing the risk of cognitive decline.

Swimming: Aquatic Option for Brain Health

How to do it

- Choose a swimming style that suits your comfort and skill level.

- Focus on controlled breathing and rhythmic movements.

Why It Is Beneficial for Memory

- Swimming is a workout that helps you with cardiovascular health.

- The buoyancy of water reduces the impact on joints, making it a suitable exercise for all ages.

- Regular swimming has been linked to improved cognitive function and mental clarity.

Cycling: Pedaling Toward Cognitive Resilience

How to do it

- Ride a bicycle outdoors or use a stationary bike.

- Start with a comfortable pace and gradually increase intensity.

- Pay attention to proper bike fit to prevent injuries.

Why It Is Beneficial for Memory

- Cycling is a low-impact cardiovascular exercise that supports brain health.

- It enhances blood flow to the brain, promoting the delivery of oxygen and nutrients.

- Regular cycling has been associated with improved cognitive performance and memory.

Balance Exercises: Stability for Cognitive Agility

How to do it

- Practice exercises that challenge balance, such as standing on one leg or using a balance board.

- Include activities like heel-to-toe walking and side-leg raises.

- Gradually increase the difficulty as your balance improves.

Why It Is Beneficial for Memory

- Balance exercises stimulate the vestibular system, crucial for spatial awareness.

- Enhanced balance contributes to fall prevention, reducing the risk of head injuries that may impact memory.

- Challenging balance activities engage cognitive processes, supporting brain health.

As you explore these exercises, keep in mind that the key to reaping the cognitive benefits of physical activity lies in consistency and enjoyment. Choose activities that align with your preferences, fitness level, and health status. Additionally, consult with healthcare professionals or fitness experts, especially if you have pre-existing health conditions.

Remember that the goal is not only physical fitness but also cognitive vitality. Whether you prefer a leisurely walk or strength training, each movement contributes to the overall well-being of your body and mind.

Nurturing Memory Through Movement

Physical exercise, even in its gentlest forms, is a valuable ally on the journey toward enhanced cognitive function and memory retention. Seniors with varying physical capabilities can still partake in exercises that are gentle yet effective. Let us explore the benefits of gentle exercises for memory improvement and guide readers in forming their own personalized exercise routine, tailored to their unique needs and preferences.

The Indirect Pathway to Memory Enhancement

Exercise, even when gentle, contributes to memory improvement through various indirect mechanisms. While the impact may not be as immediately apparent as with more intense workouts, the cumulative benefits of consistent gentle exercise are profound.

- **Improved Blood Flow to the Brain:** Gentle exercises, such as walking or tai chi, enhance blood circulation, ensuring that the brain receives an optimal supply of oxygen and nutrients. This promotes overall brain health, supporting memory functions.

- **Stress Reduction and Neurotransmitter Release:** Low-impact activities like yoga or meditation-based exercises help reduce stress and anxiety levels. In turn, this decreases the release of cortisol, a stress hormone known to negatively impact memory. Additionally, gentle exercises stimulate the release of neurotransmitters that enhance mood and cognitive function.

- **Enhanced Neuroplasticity:** Gentle exercises that involve coordination and balance, such as seated leg lifts or chair yoga, stimulate neuroplasticity. This is the brain's ability to adapt and form new connections, crucial for memory improvement.

- **Joint Mobility and Stability:** For seniors with limited physical capabilities, exercises focusing on joint mobility and stability, like seated marches or shoulder rolls, contribute to overall physical well-being. Improved joint health supports an active lifestyle, indirectly benefiting cognitive functions.

Forming an Exercise Routine for You

Creating a personalized exercise routine involves considering individual preferences, health conditions, and physical capabilities. Here is a step-by-step guide to help seniors develop their own gentle exercise routine:

- **Consult With Healthcare Professionals:** Before starting any exercise routine, especially if there are existing health concerns, consult with healthcare professionals. They can provide guidance on suitable exercises based on individual health conditions.

- **Identify Personal Preferences:** Consider activities you enjoy. Whether it is walking, seated yoga, or gentle stretching, selecting activities you find enjoyable increases the likelihood of adherence to the routine.

- **Assess Physical Capabilities:** Be honest about your current physical capabilities. Assess your strength, flexibility, and balance. This self-awareness forms the foundation for creating a routine that is both safe and effective.

- **Set Realistic Goals:** Establish achievable goals based on your current abilities. This could be as simple as increasing daily steps or incorporating gentle stretches into your routine. Setting realistic goals ensures a positive and encouraging experience.

- **Incorporate Variety:** Include a variety of exercises to address different aspects of fitness. This could involve a combination of cardiovascular exercises (e.g., seated marching), strength exercises (e.g., seated leg lifts), and flexibility exercises (e.g., gentle stretches).

- **Gradual Progression:** Start with low-intensity exercises and gradually increase the duration and intensity over time. This gradual progression minimizes the risk of injury and allows the body to adapt.

- **Adapt Exercises to Suit Your Needs:** Modify exercises based on your comfort level. If standing exercises are challenging, opt for seated variations. Use props or aids like chairs or resistance bands to provide support.

- **Incorporate Balance and Coordination Exercises:** Integrate exercises that focus on balance and coordination, such as seated leg lifts or heel-to-toe walking. These activities stimulate cognitive functions while enhancing physical stability.

- **Include Relaxation Techniques:** Dedicate time to relaxation techniques like deep breathing or mindfulness. These practices not only contribute to stress reduction but also support cognitive well-being.

- **Establish Consistency:** Consistency is key to reaping the benefits of gentle exercise. Aim for a routine that fits into your schedule, whether it is daily, a few times a week, or based on your preferences.

- **Track Progress and Adjust:** Keep a record of your exercises and how you feel after each session. Regularly assess your progress and make adjustments to the routine as needed. This ensures that your exercise plan remains aligned with your evolving capabilities and goals.

- **Stay Hydrated and Listen to Your Body:** Drink plenty of water, especially if engaging in exercises that induce mild exertion. Listen to your body's signals, and if you experience pain or discomfort beyond normal exertion, consult with healthcare professionals.

Example Gentle Exercise Routine

Here is an example of a gentle exercise routine that combines cardiovascular, strength, flexibility, and balance exercises. Remember to adapt each exercise based on your comfort level and capabilities.

Seated Marching (Cardiovascular)

- Sit comfortably in a chair.

- Lift one knee at a time in a marching motion.

- Gradually increase the pace for 5 minutes.

Seated Leg Lifts (Strength)

- Sit upright with feet flat on the floor.

- Lift one leg at a time, straightening it.

- Hold for a few seconds and lower.

- Repeat for 10 repetitions on each leg.

Gentle Arm Circles (Flexibility)

- Sit or stand comfortably.

- Extend your arms to the sides.

- Make small circular motions with your arms for 3 minutes.

Heel-to-Toe Walking (Balance and Coordination)

- Stand behind a sturdy chair for support.

- Place one foot directly in front of the other.

- Walk heel-to-toe in a straight line for 5 minutes.

Seated Forward Bend (Flexibility)

- Sit at the edge of a chair with feet flat.

- Hinge at the hips and reach toward your toes.

- Hold the stretch for 15-30 seconds.

Deep Breathing (Relaxation)

- Sit comfortably with a straight back.

- Inhale deeply through your nose for a count of four.

- Exhale slowly through pursed lips for a count of six.

- Repeat for 5 minutes.

Enjoy the process, relish the movements that bring joy, and celebrate the positive impact on both your physical and cognitive well-being. Gentle exercises, when approached with enthusiasm and consistency, become a delightful ritual that nurtures not only your memory but your overall quality of life.

As we conclude this chapter, remember that embracing a well-balanced and nourishing lifestyle is not just about physical health; it is a cornerstone for enhancing cognitive function and memory. By incorporating brain-boosting nutrients and gentle exercises, you lay the foundation for a sharper mind and a more resilient memory. In the broader framework of our quest to improve memory, this chapter serves as a crucial bridge connecting the mental and physical aspects of our well-being.

Understanding the profound impact of what we consume and how we move on our cognitive abilities empowers us to take intentional steps toward a more vibrant and enriched life. Now, armed with knowledge about brain-healthy foods and tailored exercise routines, you are better equipped to embark on a transformative journey.

In the next chapter, we will delve into the heart of the matter—overcoming memory challenges. Whether you are facing occasional forgetfulness or seeking proactive strategies to fortify your memory fortress, the next chapter will provide practical insights, proven techniques, and engaging activities to help you navigate and triumph over the hurdles that may come your way.

Chapter 8:

Overcoming Memory Challenges

You never know how much a man can't remember until he is called as a witness. –Will Rogers

Congratulations, dear reader! You have reached the final chapter of our journey together, and it is a chapter that holds the keys to overcoming memory challenges. Throughout this book, we have explored a myriad of enjoyable activities and games designed to enhance cognitive function and memory. Now, as we delve into the last chapter, we embark on a crucial phase— addressing specific memory challenges that many seniors face and uncovering effective strategies to overcome them.

Here, I will guide you through practical lifestyle changes and targeted exercises tailored to bolster your cognitive abilities. Memory concerns are a natural part of aging, but that does not mean we cannot take proactive steps to maintain and even improve our cognitive and memory capacities.

As we navigate through memory challenges, I will provide you with evidence-based insights, expert advice, and, most importantly, a toolkit of engaging activities that make the journey enjoyable. These are not just remedies; they are invitations to explore new horizons, challenge your mind, and create a lifestyle that nurtures cognitive vitality.

Remember, it is never too late to invest in your cognitive well-being, and each small change can make a significant impact.

Overcoming Specific Memory Challenges

Despite engaging with the excess of activities and games we have explored throughout this book, it is common for people to face persistent memory hurdles. Understanding these challenges is the first step toward developing targeted strategies for overcoming them. Let us delve into some of the common everyday memory challenges that you, as readers, may still be grappling with, despite your efforts.

Forgetfulness in Routine Tasks

One of the most prevalent memory challenges seniors face is forgetfulness in routine tasks. Forgetting where you placed something, whether you turned off the stove, or if you took your medication can be a source of frustration. These seemingly small lapses can accumulate and impact daily life. Fortunately, there are practical techniques to enhance recall, such as creating checklists, establishing routines, and using memory aids like reminder apps or sticky notes.

Word Retrieval Difficulties

Another common memory challenge is difficulty in recalling specific words during conversations. You might find yourself struggling to express a particular idea or remember the name of a familiar person. This can be attributed to the natural aging process affecting word retrieval. Engaging in language-based activities, such as crossword puzzles, word games, and regular conversations, can help sharpen your linguistic abilities and facilitate smoother word recall.

Prospective Memory Challenges

Prospective memory involves remembering to perform tasks in the future, like attending an appointment or taking a prescribed medication at a specific time. Seniors often encounter challenges in prospective memory, leading to missed engagements or medication lapses. Utilizing tools like alarms and calendars, and setting routine cues can significantly improve prospective memory and ensure important tasks are not overlooked.

Multitasking Difficulties

As life becomes busier, multitasking becomes inevitable. However, multitasking can strain memory, especially in older age. Juggling multiple tasks at once may result in forgetting crucial details or neglecting certain responsibilities. To overcome this challenge, it is beneficial to prioritize tasks, break them into smaller, manageable steps, and focus on one thing at a time. Additionally, mindfulness techniques can help improve attention and concentration.

Misplacing Items

Misplacing items like glasses, remote controls, or wallets is a common frustration for seniors. The "tip-of-the-tongue" phenomenon, where you know you know something but cannot quite retrieve it, is also a related issue. Implementing organizational strategies, such as designated storage spaces, can mitigate the stress of searching for misplaced items. Additionally, developing a habit of retracing your steps when searching for something can trigger memory recall.

Social Memory Challenges

Social memory challenges involve difficulty remembering names, faces, or details about people you have met. This can impact social interactions and relationships. Engaging in social activities, attending gatherings, and using mnemonic techniques like associating names with familiar objects or characteristics can aid in improving social memory.

Environmental Distractions

Seniors may find it challenging to focus and retain information in environments with excessive noise or distractions. This is particularly true when engaging in activities that require concentration, such as reading or learning new skills. Creating a quiet and organized space for cognitive activities, using noise-canceling headphones, and practicing mindfulness can enhance focus and memory retention.

Time-Related Confusion

The concept of time can become more fluid as we age, leading to confusion about dates, days of the week, or even the season. This can impact planning and scheduling. Developing a structured daily routine, using visual calendars, and incorporating time cues into your environment can provide a more concrete sense of time.

Tip-of-the-Tongue Moments

Tip-of-the-tongue moments, where you cannot immediately recall a familiar name or piece of information, are a common memory challenge. These instances can be frustrating, but they are a natural part of the aging process. Engaging in activities that stimulate memory retrieval, such as trivia games or puzzles, can help strengthen the connections in your brain responsible for these recall moments.

Technology Learning Curve

In an era dominated by technology, seniors may face challenges in learning and adapting to new devices, applications, or software. This can hinder the ability to stay connected with loved ones or engage in online activities. Taking a patient and gradual approach to technology adoption, seeking assistance when needed, and participating in technology-focused training can ease the learning curve and boost confidence.

Understanding these common memory challenges is the first step toward addressing them effectively.

General Coping Tools for Handling Memory Loss

These tools serve as foundational pillars to help you navigate the complexities of memory loss, fostering a resilient and proactive mindset. Let us explore 10 general coping tools that can empower you in your journey toward enhanced cognitive and memory capacity.

Mindfulness and Meditation

Cultivating mindfulness through meditation can be a powerful tool for managing memory challenges. Mindfulness practices promote a heightened awareness of the present moment, reducing stress and improving focus. Dedicate a few minutes each day to mindfulness exercises, such as deep breathing or guided meditation, to enhance overall cognitive well-being.

Regular Physical Exercise

Physical activity has been consistently linked to improved cognitive function and memory. Engage in regular exercise routines that suit your fitness level and preferences. Whether it is walking, swimming, yoga, or gentle aerobics, staying physically active enhances blood flow to the brain and stimulates the growth of new neurons.

Balanced Nutrition

Adopting a well-balanced and nutrient-rich diet is crucial for brain health. Include foods like fruits, vegetables, fish, and nuts. Hydration is also vital, as even mild dehydration can impact cognitive performance. It is recommended to go to a nutritionist for personalized recommendations.

Adequate Sleep

Quality sleep is essential for memory consolidation and overall cognitive function. You can start by establishing a routine aiming for 7-9 hours of uninterrupted sleep each night. If sleep disturbances persist, consult with a healthcare professional for guidance.

Social Engagement

Maintaining an active social life is not only enjoyable but also beneficial for cognitive health. Join clubs, participate in community events, or simply spend time with friends and family to foster meaningful connections.

Cognitive Stimulation

Keep your brain engaged with activities that challenge and stimulate your cognitive abilities. Puzzles, crossword games, memory exercises, and learning new skills can help create new neural connections. Incorporate a variety of mentally stimulating activities into your daily routine to keep your brain agile and adaptable.

Organization and Routine

Establishing a structured routine and maintaining an organized living space can significantly reduce memory challenges. Use calendars, planners, and reminder tools to keep track of appointments, tasks, and important dates. This not only aids memory but also provides a sense of control and reduces stress.

Stress Management Techniques

Practice stress management techniques, such as deep breathing, progressive muscle relaxation, or hobbies that bring joy and relaxation. Regularly engaging in activities that promote a sense of calmness can contribute to overall cognitive well-being.

Memory Aids and Tools

Embrace the use of memory aids and tools to support daily activities. Utilize smartphone apps, sticky notes, or digital voice recorders to jot down important information. These tools can serve as external memory extensions, helping you stay organized and remember essential details.

Regular Health Checkups

Stay proactive about your overall health by scheduling regular checkups with healthcare professionals. Conditions like hypertension, diabetes, and vitamin deficiencies can impact cognitive function. Addressing any underlying health issues on time can contribute to better memory health.

So, you see, each tool plays a unique role in promoting overall cognitive health and resilience. Now, armed with these foundational strategies, let us explore two major lifestyle changes that delve deeper into overcoming specific memory challenges. These changes are designed to enhance your cognitive abilities and elevate your quality of life.

Sleeping Right for Enhanced Memory

Sleep is not merely a period of rest; it is a critical process that plays a fundamental role in memory consolidation and overall brain health. As we explore the impact of sleep on memory, we will unravel the intricate relationship between a good night's sleep and the enhancement of cognitive abilities.

Memory Consolidation

Sleep is often referred to as the brain's filing system. Throughout the day, our brains accumulate a vast amount of information and experiences. It is during sleep, particularly during the deep stages of non-REM (rapid eye movement) sleep, that this information is processed and consolidated into long-term memories.

During these stages, the brain undergoes a complex dance of neural activity, strengthening the connections between neurons associated with the newly acquired information. This consolidation process is crucial for transforming short-term memories into more permanent forms, making them easier to retrieve later.

Learning Enhancement

High-quality sleep not only solidifies existing memories but also enhances the ability to learn new information. Research suggests that individuals who enjoy sufficient and restorative sleep are better equipped to grasp new concepts, acquire new skills, and retain information for longer periods.

The benefits extend beyond academic or work-related learning; they encompass the acquisition of new hobbies and languages and even the mastery of various cognitive activities that we have explored throughout this book.

Emotional Regulation

Sleep plays a pivotal role in emotional well-being and regulation. Adequate sleep helps to regulate mood and stress levels, which, in turn, can impact memory. Emotional experiences are often intertwined with memory formation, and quality sleep aids in processing and contextualizing these experiences.

Lack of sleep, on the other hand, can contribute to heightened emotional reactivity and increased susceptibility to stress, potentially impacting memory recall and overall cognitive function.

Synaptic Plasticity

Synaptic plasticity, the ability of synapses (the connections between neurons) to strengthen or weaken over time, is a key component of memory formation. Sleep supports this process by influencing the balance of neurotransmitters and facilitating the removal of unnecessary information.

Adequate sleep enhances synaptic plasticity, allowing the brain to adapt to new information and experiences. This adaptability is essential for maintaining a sharp and flexible memory.

The Pillars of High-Quality Sleep

Now that we understand the profound impact of sleep on memory, let us delve into the essential components of achieving high-quality sleep.

Consistent Sleep Schedule

Establishing a consistent sleep schedule helps regulate the body's internal clock, optimizing the quality of your sleep. Aim to go to bed and wake up at the same time every day, even on weekends. This consistency reinforces the natural circadian rhythm, promoting more restful sleep.

Create a Relaxing Bedtime Routine

Engage in calming activities before bedtime to signal to your body that it is time to wind down. This could include reading a book, practicing relaxation techniques, or taking a warm bath. Avoid stimulating activities, such as watching intense television shows or using electronic devices, at least an hour before bedtime.

Optimize Sleep Environment

Create a sleep-conducive environment in your bedroom. Keep the room cool, dark, and quiet. Invest in a comfortable mattress and pillows that support a restful night's sleep. Remove electronic devices that emit light and consider using blackout curtains to minimize external disturbances.

Limit Stimulants and Heavy Meals

Limit the intake of substances such as caffeine and nicotine, especially in the hours leading up to bedtime. Also, avoid heavy meals.

Regular Exercise

Regular physical activity contributes to better sleep quality. You can go for a walk for at least 30 minutes. However, avoid heavy exercise since it may have a stimulating effect.

Mindfulness and Relaxation Techniques

Incorporate these techniques into your daily routine. Practices such as deep breathing, meditation, or gentle yoga can promote relaxation, reduce stress, and prepare your mind for restful sleep.

Limit Naps

While short naps can be rejuvenating, long or irregular napping during the day can interfere with nighttime sleep. If you need to nap, aim for a short duration (20-30 minutes) and avoid napping late in the afternoon.

Manage Stress

Chronic stress can be a significant barrier to quality sleep. Implement stress management techniques, such as journaling, talking to a friend, or engaging in hobbies you enjoy. By addressing stressors in your life, you pave the way for a more peaceful and restorative sleep.

Limit Screen Time

Limit screen time before bedtime, and consider using "night mode" settings on devices or wearing blue light-blocking glasses in the evening.

Seek Professional Help if Needed

If persistent sleep issues disrupt your daily life, consider seeking advice from a healthcare professional. Sleep disorders, such as insomnia or sleep apnea, can significantly impact the quality of your sleep and may require specialized intervention.

In conclusion, high-quality sleep is not just a necessity for physical health; it is a cornerstone for maintaining and enhancing cognitive abilities, particularly memory. By prioritizing consistent and restorative sleep, you empower your brain to efficiently process information, consolidate memories, and adapt to new challenges.

As we continue our exploration of overcoming memory challenges, remember that the journey to a sharper memory begins with a good night's sleep. It is a simple yet potent strategy that sets the stage for the lifestyle changes we will explore in the next sections.

Sleep Hygiene Tips for Improved Mental Well-being

Opt for a Comfortable Sleep Position

Experiment with different sleep positions to find one that provides comfort and supports spinal alignment. Using supportive pillows for your head and between your knees, if needed, can contribute to a more restful sleep.

Invest in Comfortable Bedding

Choose comfortable sheets and blankets that regulate temperature and create a cozy sleep environment. The goal is to create a bed that invites you to relax and unwind.

Address Sleep Disruptions Promptly

If you experience persistent sleep disruptions, such as snoring, insomnia, or restless legs, address them promptly. Consult with a healthcare professional to identify and address any underlying issues. Seeking timely intervention can contribute to improved sleep quality and overall mental well-being.

Practice Relaxation Techniques

Incorporate relaxation techniques into your bedtime routine. Practices such as progressive muscle relaxation, deep breathing, or guided imagery can help calm your mind and prepare your body for restful sleep.

Create a Sleep-Inducing Atmosphere

Engage your senses to create a sleep-inducing atmosphere. Use calming scents, such as lavender, in the bedroom. Consider playing soft, soothing music or white noise to drown out potential disturbances. These sensory cues can signal to your brain that it is time to unwind.

Limit Napping, If Necessary

While short naps can be rejuvenating, excessive daytime napping may interfere with nighttime sleep. If you find yourself needing to nap frequently, consider adjusting your sleep schedule or exploring other relaxation techniques to address daytime fatigue.

Mindfulness Meditation for Sleep

Mindfulness meditation, particularly tailored for sleep, can be a powerful tool. Apps and guided meditations designed for sleep can assist in quieting the mind and promoting a tranquil mental state conducive to quality sleep.

Track Your Sleep Patterns

Tracking your sleep can help identify trends, potential disruptions, and patterns that may be impacting the quality of your rest. Share this information with healthcare professionals if seeking guidance on sleep-related concerns.

Incorporating these sleep habits and hygiene tips into your routine can contribute to improved mental well-being and, consequently, enhance your memory. Remember that the goal is not just to sleep but to sleep well—to create an environment that nurtures restorative sleep and supports your cognitive vitality.

Stress Management for Enhanced Memory

In the intricate dance of memory and cognitive function, stress can play a disruptive role, affecting both the formation and retrieval of memories. As we explore the relationship between stress and memory, it becomes evident that managing stress is not only beneficial for mental well-being but is also a key factor in overcoming memory challenges.

How Stress Impacts Memory Loss

- **Hippocampus Vulnerability:** The hippocampus, a region of the brain crucial for memory formation and retrieval, is particularly vulnerable to the effects of stress. Chronic stress can lead to changes in the structure and function of the hippocampus, impairing its ability to create and store memories effectively.

- **Cortisol Overload:** Stress triggers the release of cortisol, a hormone associated with the body's fight-or-flight response. While cortisol is essential for survival in acute situations, prolonged exposure, as seen in chronic stress, can have detrimental effects on memory. Elevated cortisol levels can interfere with synaptic regulation and impair the consolidation of new memories.

- **Impact on Attention and Focus:** Stress can divert attention and focus away from the task at hand, making it challenging to encode and recall information. Individuals experiencing stress may find it difficult to concentrate, which can contribute to memory lapses and forgetfulness.

- **Influence on Memory Retrieval:** Stress can also impact the retrieval of stored memories. It may lead to a heightened state of arousal, making it challenging to recall information accurately. This phenomenon is commonly known as "stress-induced retrieval impairment."

How Memory Loss Worsens Stress

- **Cognitive Strain:** Experiencing memory challenges can create cognitive strain, adding an extra layer of stress to daily life. Forgetting important details, appointments, or names may lead to frustration and a sense of helplessness, amplifying overall stress levels.

- **Social and Emotional Impact:** Memory loss can affect social interactions and relationships. Forgetting names, faces, or shared experiences may lead to feelings of isolation and anxiety. The emotional toll of these experiences can contribute to elevated stress levels.

- **Fear of Cognitive Decline:** The fear of cognitive decline itself can be a significant stressor. Worries about memory lapses and the potential progression of cognitive challenges can create a cycle of stress that further exacerbates memory difficulties.

Stress Management Techniques

Now that we have explored the intricate relationship between stress and memory, let us delve into effective stress management techniques tailored for seniors. These techniques not only contribute to a more serene and balanced mental state but also play a pivotal role in overcoming memory challenges.

- **Deep Breathing Exercises:** Deep breathing exercises, such as diaphragmatic breathing or box breathing, can activate the body's relaxation response. Practice these techniques regularly to calm the nervous system, reduce stress hormones, and promote a sense of mental clarity.

- **Mindfulness Meditation:** Mindfulness meditation involves bringing attention to the present moment without judgment. Incorporate mindfulness into your routine through guided meditations, mindful breathing, or mindful walking. This practice enhances self-awareness and resilience in the face of stressors.

- **Progressive Muscle Relaxation (PMR):** PMR involves systematically tensing and then relaxing different muscle groups. This technique helps release physical tension and promotes relaxation. Regular practice can contribute to a reduction in overall stress levels.

- **Engage in Relaxing Hobbies:** Pursue hobbies that bring joy and relaxation. Whether it is reading, gardening, painting, or listening to music, engaging in activities you love provides a healthy escape from stressors and fosters a positive mental state.

- **Social Connection:** Meaningful conversations, shared experiences, and a robust support system can act as buffers against stress. Social engagement is a powerful tool for emotional well-being.

- **Regular Physical Exercise:** Exercise not only benefits physical health but is also a potent stress reliever. Engage in regular physical activity, choosing activities that bring enjoyment and suit your fitness level. Exercise releases endorphins, the body's natural mood lifters.

- **Cognitive Behavioral Techniques:** Work with a mental health professional to learn and apply these techniques to manage stress, reduce anxiety, and promote a positive mindset.

- **Laugh and Find Humor:** Laughter is a natural stress reliever. Watch a comedy, share jokes with friends, or attend a live performance. Finding moments of joy and humor in everyday life can contribute to a more resilient and stress-resistant mindset.

- **Establish a Daily Routine:** Creating a structured daily routine provides a sense of predictability and control. Plan your day, including dedicated time for relaxation, hobbies, and social interactions. A well-organized routine can reduce the chaos and stress often associated with uncertainty.

- **Professional Support:** If stress becomes overwhelming or persistent, seeking support from a mental health professional can be invaluable. Therapy, counseling, or stress management programs tailored to your individual needs can provide effective coping strategies and emotional guidance.

Incorporating these stress management techniques into your daily life not only fosters improved mental well-being but also contributes to a more favorable environment for memory enhancement. By adopting these techniques, you empower yourself to navigate the complexities of memory enhancement with resilience, joy, and a clearer mental focus.

In this chapter, we explored the intricate relationship between sleep, stress, and memory, uncovering the important role these factors play in shaping our cognitive abilities. By understanding the impact of high-quality sleep and effective stress management on memory, we have laid the groundwork for a comprehensive approach to overcoming memory challenges. This serves as a bridge, connecting the dots between lifestyle choices, mental well-being, and the ultimate goal of enhancing memory. As we move forward in our journey, armed with proven strategies and a deeper understanding, we are better equipped to embrace a lifestyle that not only sharpens our memory but also fosters a fulfilling and resilient cognitive vitality in the golden years.

Conclusion

In conclusion, dear readers, our journey together has been one of discovery, empowerment, and joy. Throughout this book, we have explored the fascinating world of cognitive health for seniors, debunking myths and revealing the true potential within each of you.

The main message is clear: Age may bring its challenges, but it also opens the door to exciting opportunities for cognitive enhancement. Remember, it is never too late to start exercising your brain and embracing a lifestyle that nurtures cognitive well-being.

We delved into the science of aging brains, understanding that change is a natural part of life. Then we celebrated the power of nutrition and lifestyle, emphasizing the importance of a well-balanced diet and regular physical activity. I also introduced you to the world of brain games and puzzles, proving that mental workouts can be both enjoyable and beneficial.

You have explored the significance of social connections, highlighting the positive impact of engaging with friends and loved ones. And finally, I showcased the importance of mindfulness and relaxation techniques, providing a holistic approach to cognitive well-being.

As we close this chapter of our shared journey, let me leave you with a heartening success. Now, armed with the knowledge gained from these pages, I encourage you to embark on your own journey toward cognitive vitality. Your memory can be as sharp as a T.A.C.K. (Thoughtful, Active, Curious, and Knowledgeable) with the application of these proven tools. Make them a part of your daily routine, revisit them often, and watch as your cognitive abilities flourish.

I invite you to share your own success stories and insights with the community, fostering a supportive environment for continued growth. Your experiences are valuable, and they have the potential to inspire others on their journey.

Before we part ways, I kindly ask for your feedback. Your thoughts and reviews are essential in helping others discover the benefits of these pages. Together, let us create a community dedicated to thriving cognitive health in our golden years.

Thank you for joining me on this enriching exploration. May your days be filled with curiosity, laughter, and the joy of a sharp and resilient mind.

References

Age-related memory loss. (n.d.). Retrieved February 27, 2024, from https://www.helpguide.org/articles/alzheimers-dementia-aging/age-related-memory-loss.htm#:~:text=The%20hippocampus%2C%20a%20region%2

Babaei, P., & Azari, H. B. (2022). Exercise training improves memory performance in older adults: A narrative review of evidence and possible mechanisms. *ProQuest, 15.* https://doi.org/10.3389/fnhum.2021.771553

The benefit of puzzles for the brain. (2023). Progress Lifeline. https://www.progresslifeline.org.uk/news/the-benefit-of-puzzles-for-the-brain#:~:text=Puzzles%20increase%20the%20production%20of

Bertacchi, D. (2020, August 28). *DIY memory game cards for kids (free printable).* StlMotherhood. https://stlmotherhood.com/make-your-own-memory-game-free-printable/

Bertrand, E. (2023). *Maximize memory function with a nutrient-rich diet.* Mayo Clinic Health System.

https://www.mayoclinichealthsystem.org/hom
etown-health/speaking-of-health/maximize-
memory-function-with-a-nutrient-rich-
diet#:~:text=Dark%2C%20leafy%20greens%2
0are%20known

Bomb, M. (2024). *Rebus collection 5*. Mental Bomb.
https://mentalbomb.com/rebus-collection-5/

Brain-boosting recipes. (n.d.). BBC Good Food.
https://www.bbcgoodfood.com/recipes/collec
tion/brain-boosting-recipes

Brysha, D. (2021). *Feeling stuck? Try these 18 journal
prompts for clarity*.
https://myselfcaresociety.com/blog/feeling-
stuck-try-these-18-journal-prompts-to-gain-
clarity/

Cam, D. (2023). *13 ways to improve mental math skills*.
WikiHow.
https://www.wikihow.com/Improve-Mental-
Math-Skills

Caregiver guide: Memory problems. (2015).
HealthinAging.org.
https://www.healthinaging.org/tools-and-
tips/caregiver-guide-memory-problems

Conditions. (n.d.). Retrieved February 27, 2024, from
https://myhealth.alberta.ca/Health/Pages/con
ditions.aspx?hwi

Coping with memory loss. (2022, May 6). Alzheimer's Society. https://www.alzheimers.org.uk/get-support/staying-independent/coping-with-memory-loss#:~:text=Set%20up%20a%20regular%20daily

Dana Sullivan Killroy. (2014, September 8). *Exercise plan for seniors.* Healthline; Healthline Media. https://www.healthline.com/health/everyday-fitness/senior-workouts

Delgado, J. (2023, February 23). *Can meditation improve attention, memory, and cognition?* Virginian Rehabilitation & Wellness. https://www.vaoptherapy.org/new-blog/can-meditation-improve-attention-memory-and-cognitionnbsp#:~:text=Regular%20meditation%20increases%20blood

The differences between normal aging and dementia. (n.d.). Alzheimer Society of Canada. https://alzheimer.ca/en/about-dementia/do-i-have-dementia/differences-between-normal-aging-dementia#:~:text=Some%20of%20us%20will%20experience

The emotional impact of living with memory loss. (2021). Www.alzheimers.org.uk. https://www.alzheimers.org.uk/about-

dementia/symptoms-and-
diagnosis/symptoms/emotions-memory-
loss#:~:text=They%20may%20begin%20to%2
0withdraw

A good night's sleep. (n.d.). National Institute on Aging.
https://www.nia.nih.gov/health/sleep/good-
nights-sleep

Harvard Health Publishing. (2017, March 20). *Stress relief tips for older adults.* Harvard Health; Harvard Health.
https://www.health.harvard.edu/stress/stress-
relief-tips-for-older-adults

Harvard Health Publishing. (2021, February 12).
Forgetfulness — 7 types of normal memory problems - Harvard Health. Harvard Health; Harvard
Health. https://www.health.harvard.edu/mind-
and-mood/forgetfulness-7-types-of-normal-
memory-problems

Haupt, A. (2022, February 10). Losing your keys doesn't mean you're losing your mind. Here's how to find your stuff. *Washington Post.*
https://www.washingtonpost.com/wellness/20
22/02/10/how-to-stop-losing-things/

How to create a daily routine to benefit seniors. (n.d.). Amy's
Helping   Hands.
https://www.amyshelpinghands.ca/family-

caregiver-tips-134/how-to-create-a-daily-routine-to-benefit-seniors

Hwang, J., Park, S., & Kim, S. (2018). Effects of participation in social activities on cognitive function among middle-aged and older adults in Korea. *International Journal of Environmental Research and Public Health*, *15*(10), 2315. https://doi.org/10.3390/ijerph15102315

Jjavaid. (2024, February 4). *Healthy aging: Brain health in the elderly.* Solutions Waves. https://solutionswaves.com/healthy-aging-brain-health-in-the-elderly/

Karim, H. (2024). *25 gentle exercises for seniors at home | Lottie.* Lottie.org. https://lottie.org/care-guides/exercises-for-seniors-at-home/

Kautzer, K. (2018, May 23). *22 writing prompts about childhood memories.* WriteShop. https://writeshop.com/blog/writing-prompts-about-childhood-memories/

Kwik, J. (2023, February 24). *10 brain reasons to make reading a habit.* Medium. https://kwikbrain.medium.com/10-brain-reasons-to-make-reading-a-habit-aa628d4b498c

LaMotte, S. (2023, December 26). *How to reduce your risk of early-onset dementia, according to science.* CNN.

https://edition.cnn.com/2023/12/26/health/e
arly-dementia-risk-study-wellness/index.html

Lighthouse School. (2021, April 23). *Create your own DIY memory match game for kids.* https://www.lighthousewillis.com/blog/craft-ideas/create-your-own-diy-memory-match-game-for-kids/

LinkedIn Community. (n.d.). *What are the best memory games to play with your team for fun and learning?* Retrieved February 27, 2024, from https://www.linkedin.com/advice/0/what-best-memory-games-play-your-team-fun

Mayo Clinic Staff. (2019). *Memory loss: 7 tips to improve your memory.* Mayo Clinic. https://www.mayoclinic.org/healthy-lifestyle/healthy-aging/in-depth/memory-loss/art-20046518

Mayo Clinic Staff. (2022). *When you should seek help for memory loss.* Mayo Clinic. https://www.mayoclinic.org/diseases-conditions/alzheimers-disease/in-depth/memory-loss/art-20046326#:~:text=Everyone%20forgets%20thi ngs%20at%20ti

Melone, L. (2015, April 16). *10 brain exercises that boost memory.* Everyday Health.

https://www.everydayhealth.com/longevity/m
ental-fitness/brain-exercises-for-memory.aspx

Memories. (n.d.). Retrieved February 27, 2024, from
https://memories.net/blog/how-to-overcome-
the-fear-of-forgetting-a-loved-one

Memory problems, forgetfulness, and aging. (2023). National
Institute on Aging.
https://www.nia.nih.gov/health/memory-loss-
and-forgetfulness/memory-problems-
forgetfulness-and-aging#:~:text=It'

Memory: Myth versus truth. (2021, November 15). John
Hopkins Medicine.
https://www.hopkinsmedicine.org/health/well
ness-and-prevention/memory-myth-versus-
truth#:~:text=Myth%3A%20Forgetfulness%20
%3D%20Alzheimer'

Mendel, B. (2017, August 29). *Does meditation improve
memory?* Mindworks.
https://mindworks.org/blog/does-meditation-
improve-
memory/#:~:text=Simply%20put%2C%20min
dfulness%20meditation%20(

Metivier, A. (2021, June 30). *Magnetic memory method -
memory improvement made easy.* Magnetic Memory
Method.
https://www.magneticmemorymethod.com/ho
w-to-remember-conversations/

Miller, M. (2019). *Inside the science of memory.* John Hopkins Medicine. https://www.hopkinsmedicine.org/wellness-and-prevention/inside-the-science-of-memory

Mohs, R. (2007, May 17). *How to improve your memory.* HowStuffWorks. https://health.howstuffworks.com/human-body/systems/nervous-system/how-to-improve-your-memory4.htm#:~:text=Use%20all%20your%20senses.

Myths about dementia, alzheimers and memory loss. (2020). Cedars-Sinai. https://www.cedars-sinai.org/blog/dementia-alzheimers-and-memory-loss.html

National Institutes of Health. (2017, July 13). *Sleep on it.* NIH News in Health. https://newsinhealth.nih.gov/2013/04/sleep-it

NIH. (2023). *Memory problems, forgetfulness and aging.* National Institute on Aging. https://www.nia.nih.gov/health/memory-loss-and-forgetfulness/memory-problems-forgetfulness-and-aging#:~:text=Getting%20lost%20in%20places%20you

Online memory matching game for adults: Symbols. (n.d.). Free Memory Games Online for Adults. Retrieved February 27, 2024, from https://www.tucogames.com/memory-games/30-memory-for-adults.html

Pahadia, A. (2023, June 20). *101 memories quotes to embrace the beautiful moments in life.* PINKVILLA. https://www.pinkvilla.com/lifestyle/relationships/memories-quotes-1226439

Pawlik-Kienlen, L. (2022). *Ways to boost your memory.* Health. https://www.health.com/condition/alzheimers/15-ways-to-boost-your-memory-in-your-30s-40s-50s-and-beyond#:~:text=In%20fact%2C%20experts%20say%20you

Penn Medicine. (2020, December 31). *The 7 stages of Alzheimer's disease.* Www.pennmedicine.org. https://www.pennmedicine.org/updates/blogs/neuroscience-blog/2019/november/stages-of-alzheimers

Protect your brain from stress. (2018, August 1). Harvard Health. https://www.health.harvard.edu/mind-and-mood/protect-your-brain-from-stress#:~:text=

Reese, H. (2022). A neurologist's tips to protect your memory. *The New York Times.*

https://www.nytimes.com/2022/07/06/well/mind/memory-loss-prevention.html

Roberts, K. (2014). *Knowing a child's learning style improves memory skills.* Www.psychologytoday.com. https://www.psychologytoday.com/us/blog/savvy-parenting/201403/knowing-child-s-learning-style-improves-memory-skills#:~:text=Auditory%20learners%20hear%20the%20informa

Sapega, S. (2017, January 30). *Playing an instrument: Better for your brain than just listening.* Penn Medicine News. https://www.pennmedicine.org/news/news-blog/2017/january/playing-an-instrument-better-for-your-brain-than-just-listening

Shebek, S. (2022, October 18). *ZZZs please: New research shows how to boost memory during sleep.* University of UTAH Health. https://uofuhealth.utah.edu/newsroom/news/2022/10/zzzs-please-new-research-shows-how-boost-memory-during-sleep

Sikowski, S. (2019, October 9). *How to use a planner effectively.* Herzing University. https://www.herzing.edu/blog/how-use-planner-effectively

Stanborough, R. J. (2020, October 19). *10 benefits of playing chess: Plus potential downsides.* Healthline.

https://www.healthline.com/health/benefits-of-playing-chess

10 word games to train your brain. (n.d.). Retrieved February 27, 2024, from https://www.readlax.com/blog/en/word_games_train_brain

Umberson, D., & Karas Montez, J. (2011). Social relationships and health: A flashpoint for health policy. *Journal of Health and Social Behavior, 51*(1), 54–66. https://doi.org/10.1177/0022146510383501

University of Central Florida. (n.d.). *9 types of mnemonics for better memory.* https://www.seattleu.edu/media/learning-assistance-programs/files/9-Types-of-Mnemonics-for-Better-Memorya4b4.pdf

Image References

Brooke Lark. (2017). *Variedad de frutas en rodajas.* [Image]. Unsplash. https://unsplash.com/es/fotos/variedad-de-frutas-en-rodajas-08bOYnH_r_E

Clker-Free-Vector-Images. (2012). Imagen de Memoria, Tarjeta y Bordo. [Image]. Pixabay.

https://pixabay.com/es/vectors/memoria-tarjeta-bordo-juego-48118/

Cottonbro Studio. (2021). *Amigos mujer jugando adentro.* [Image]. Pexels. https://www.pexels.com/es-es/foto/amigos-mujer-jugando-adentro-6939465/

Leloo the First. (2020). *Simple Motivacional Contra Dudas.* [Image]. Pexels. https://www.pexels.com/es-es/foto/inscripcion-simple-motivacional-contra-dudas-5238645/https://www.pexels.com/es-es/foto/inscripcion-simple-motivacional-contra-dudas-5238645/

Mike Murray. (2020). *Planificador Vista Superior.* [Image]. Pexels. https://www.pexels.com/es-es/foto/naturaleza-muerta-planificador-vista-superior-clips-de-la-carpeta-6446238/

OpenClipart-Vectors. (2013). *Imagen de As, Tarjetas y Club.* [Image]. Pixabay. https://pixabay.com/es/vectors/as-tarjetas-club-diamante-corazón-159856/

Randy Fath. (2018). *Fotografía de enfoque selectivo de piezas de ajedrez.* [Image]. Unsplash. https://unsplash.com/es/fotos/fotografia-de-enfoque-selectivo-de-piezas-de-ajedrez-G1yhU1Ej-9A

Tumisu. (2018). *Imagen de Salud mental, Mental y Salud. De uso gratuito.* [Image]. Pixabay. https://pixabay.com/es/illustrations/salud-mental-mental-salud-cabeza-3337026/

Unsplash+. (2022). *Foto del entrenamiento de la función de la mano del paciente masculino con accidente cerebrovascular mediante el uso de un....*[Image]. Unsplash. https://unsplash.com/es/fotos/foto-del-entrenamiento-de-la-funcion-de-la-mano-del-paciente-masculino-con-accidente-cerebrovascular-mediante-el-uso-de-un-tablero-perforado-de-varios-colores-en-la-sala-de-terapia-en-el-hospital-HmiWTvxgBzQ

Made in United States
Orlando, FL
20 April 2025

60648001R00148